Courage
in
Cannabis

Presented By
Dr. Bridget Cole Williams, MD

Acknowledgements

Thank you to our sponsors for giving a voice to cannabis stories.

Emerald Sponsor

Compass Natural
Endo Vibe Cannabis Center
Spendr
Supherbs
The Canna Mom Show

Jade Sponsor

BLEV 614 Network
CannabisBPO
Columbus Botanical Depot
Dagga Digital Marketing
Hemp Box Etc.
Ohio Medical Marijuana Physicians Association

See the Sponsor Profiles in the back of the book

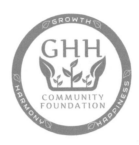

Courage in Cannabis book series is a project of the GHH Community Foundation, a 501(c)(3) nonprofit. To support the book series development, become an author, donate or sponsor; learn more at: www.courageincannabis.com

Learn more about Courage in Cannabis and the GHH Community Foundation at:
www.courageincannabis.org

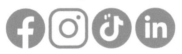

@CourageinCannBooks

"Every noteworthy person has a story of adversity
they had to overcome to become great.
The power is not in the hardship they endured,
the power is in the COURAGE they gathered to defy it."

-Dr. Bridget Cole Williams, MD

Amongst the chapters you will see quotes and short testimonials from impactful voices in the cannabis space. These are our "sparks". These individuals are defining courage, influencing our opinions and setting fire to the cannabis movement.

Table of Contents

Foreword

By Adam Wilks

Words are meaningful. Perception is powerful. Today, what we call cannabis and what has grown to become over a sixteen billion dollar per year industry has changed lives both physically and economically. But before there was a cannabis global empire, there was a fourteen-year-old me, smoking weed for fun, relaxation, creativity, socially or just because.

Smoking weed socially as a young teen was not uncommon among my peers. We were not bad kids. We were just curious young men and products of our environment. It was just there. A part of my life. Something I enjoyed. It was also something I learned.

Weed. That's what we called it. Books and ads telling us to stay away from it called it marijuana. Our parents called it reefer. Police who threw young boys in jail for carrying it called it dope. Now, business executives call it cannabis. But at fourteen, it was regular old weed, and I knew the world would view my smoking as a negative thing. But I never understood why.

Even when I was young and uneducated, I understood that weed was natural and from the earth. I didn't understand the negative connotations surrounding it, and I was too naïve to know that wordplay, perceptions, research, business models, and paid taxes would one day transform my teenage recreation into a legal, thriving, and profitable enterprise.

With my contacts and access to it, I naturally became the plug for my friends, classmates, and neighborhood. I also got a glimpse of its earning potential and money management.

At age seventeen, my experience with weed evolved even more, and I was forever changed. The rock and soul of our family, my dear grandmother, was diagnosed with brain cancer. Her brain tumor was aggressive, and she was on numerous pain medications to help her cope with the tremendous pain that invaded her body. One day, I saw her looking weak, physically drained, and honestly, defeated. She softly asked me to give her a joint. I was shocked. Not just that my grandmother had asked me for weed, but stunned that she was seeking some type of comfort from this simple herb.

On the dresser next to her, there were more medications than I could count, all with names I would not even try to pronounce. She began to smoke, and instantly her body seemed more relaxed. I know you can't see peace, but at that moment, I saw her peace. She was comfortable.

Weed tremendously reducing her pain was the first experience and proof I had that showed me this is not just a simple little herb that can generate a calming buzz. Weed has healing and relief properties, and I would never forget it. As an adult, I became more interested in educating myself on what formulas, amounts, and presentations of weed were the most effective and safe for healing. I became even more critical of the criminalization of it and wanted to better understand the root of why it was still socially and legally frowned upon. The answer was the lack of education and control. We, as a society, do not approve of what we don't understand. I became vested in understanding and regurgitating to others what I learned.

In the words of Gandhi, "Each one, teach one."

In my learning and understanding, these things became clear:

- Cannabis undoubtedly has healing power.
- It is the most powerful herb on the planet.
- It can help those addicted to narcotics to be released from those drugs.
- It can lower blood pressure.
- It can help fight cancer.
- It calms anxiety.

It temporarily quiets an overstimulated, busy mind. Ironically, for decades we were bamboozled into not questioning the belief that marijuana was a gateway drug that leads to harsher drugs when in reality, it presents a safe option to eliminate or never even begin other drugs.* Cannabis is a miracle plant-based drug. When sourced legally and ethically, it is safe. Even more rigorously and effectively tested than the fruits and vegetables we eat.

Anxiolytics and opioid addiction are widespread and ruining countless lives in our country. I personally have had to check family members into rehab, and it is a painful experience that I never want to relive or wish upon anyone. Cannabis is proven to medically ease pain and anxiety and could and should be introduced as an option versus these other harsh and dangerous drugs.

There is power in cannabis.

I went on to become a business executive with expertise in licensing and franchising in other industries, but I never forgot the power of cannabis. I believed in it so much that I have now been involved in over thirty cannabis brands, and when I met boxing legend Mike Tyson and business executive Chad

Bronstein, they were seeking a CEO with extensive cannabis expertise and asked me to jump in. I was happy to do so.

My once side hustle has become a successful career in a thriving industry. As the CEO of Tyson 2.0, I have had the pleasure of reimagining the brand that Mike Tyson brilliantly envisioned. Under my leadership, Tyson 2.0 has expanded to over twenty-five states and three countries. We have also secured over fifteen million dollars in funding and led the company in over one hundred million dollars worth of distribution deals. What does this success mean? It means that times have changed, and knowledge paired with authentic branding and an exceptional team is supreme.

Medical marijuana use is widely accepted and recreationally legal in nineteen states and medically legal in thirty-seven states.* Companies that earn millions of dollars in revenue per year in cannabis sales, distributing thousands of pounds of cannabis, are celebrated and recognized. But I, as a business leader and simply an empathetic human, can't stop there.

Much has changed with the perception of what we now almost solely refer to as cannabis, although this change did not happen soon enough. And there is still work to do. We have upgraded the name and packaging, but negative connotations still exist socially and, more importantly, legally.

Throughout the last few decades, more emphasis has been placed on weed as an uncontrolled, criminal substance. Marijuana arrests make up over half of all drug arrests in America.* And many of those arrested are still serving time. Nationwide, these arrests are proven to be racially biased, with Black men being almost four times more likely to be convicted for possessing marijuana than non-Blacks.* As much as I appreciate the upward trend in the business of cannabis, if we as a society can align on the power of cannabis, we can also admit that the past and current criminalization of cannabis is flawed.

Where do we go from here? We educate, advocate, and serve. We educate our friends, family, and even our children on what cannabis is and what it isn't. We must educate on safe cannabis uses and warn of the dangerous non tested street products. We look negativity and judgment in the face and replace them with education. We advocate when the opportunity presents itself for those who are being judged or criminalized for cannabis use. We speak up and urge our elected officials to stop treating cannabis use and minor distribution as violent crimes. And for those we care for who sell on the streets, we must encourage them to think bigger. We must let them know that hustles can become empires. And for those of us who are cannabis executives, we must serve. We have a responsibility to see beyond the bottom line and growing success and remember that to whom much is given, much is required. For me, this means both charity and creating a path of success for others. For me, the power of cannabis is the healing properties it has, the legal business opportunities it makes obtainable, and the options it provides current or would-be addicts.

I hope we continue to de-stigmatize cannabis and that the next generation, which includes my amazing sons Jake Stone Wilks and Dylan Beau Wilks, will be knowledgeable and make safe, informed decisions, and be able to differentiate between cannabis myths and facts.

What about you? Have you discovered the power of cannabis?

My hope for you, the reader, is that you are encouraged by the impactful stories and testimonies that you are about to experience in this book and get inspired to gain your own knowledge and understanding of this miracle plant.

There is power in cannabis, and power is knowledge. This power is yours.

Statistics

https://www.aclu.org/gallery/marijuana-arrests-numbers

https://www.jwu.edu/news/2021/09/7-potential-health-benefits-of-cannabis.html

https://www.fox9.com/news/marijuana-laws-by-us-state-2022

https://www.independent.co.uk/life-style/health-and-families/study-marijuana-hard-drugsprevent-gateway-study-addiction-jacob-miguel-vigil-new-mexico-a7960616.html?amp

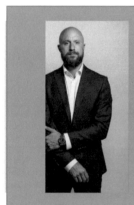

Adam Wilks
CEO of Tyson 2.0
www.tyson20.com

Learn more about Adam at
www.courageincannabis.com:

"Cannabis has been a major component in my health and wellness routine. The healing I receive on a mental and physical level has greatly improved the quality of my life. This book is a must read for those interested in learning more about the wonderful holistic healing benefits available through the marijuana plant."

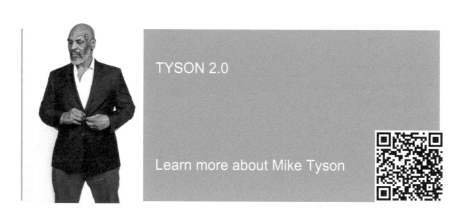

TYSON 2.0

Learn more about Mike Tyson

My All-American Cannabis Story

By Gerald A. Moore Jr.

My All-American cannabis story began in 2006 while hanging out with a group of high school friends at a social gathering consuming cannabis. This night changed my life and perspective on the cannabis plant and society because I felt like so many people had deceived me. Cannabis made me feel amazing, and most of the things I was told were not one hundred percent accurate.

At the time, cannabis was illegal in Maryland, but like many high school students, I was at the age of experimentation and challenging the rules.

Growing up in the late 90s and early 2000s, I was practically driven into fear over cannabis through school programs like D.A.R.E. and the Just Say No marketing campaigns. My house was a dry home even though, in my early years, my grandfather was a alcohol drinker, cannabis consumer, and cultivator which I found out in my thirties from my aunts.

From as far back as I can remember, I was told that if I wanted to be a successful in life and pursue an athletic career I needed to stay away from drugs and alcohol.

I was a highly recruited two-sport athlete in high school. I attended St. Johns College High School, a prestigious college preparatory school in the nation's capital, Washington, DC, which is one of the most competitive high school sports conferences in the country.

My high school environment was intense, very political, and bougie. This environment came with a lot of anxiety and stress especially being an outsider. There was tremendous pressure to be a high achiever with grades and to perform athletically. Growing up Black in the spotlight and in a privileged educational environment made it much more challenging to navigate life. For me, it was difficult to navigate sober.

I often felt out of place because I did not come from a well-off family like many of my peers. However, my athleticism and my parent's ability to break into the middle class afforded me the opportunity to become involved in various academic, social, and athletic situations that most people in my family had never experienced.

I noticed early on in my encounters with cannabis that it helped me to relax and also helped with my aches and pains from sports. By the time my junior year came around, I was being recruited by major and mid-level Division 1 universities nationally. However, being that I was not too concerned with attending big universities, I verbally committed to Ohio University during my junior year and signed my national letter of intent in 2008, my senior year.

Two weeks after graduating high school, my parents dropped me off in Athens, Ohio, for summer school.

If you are unfamiliar with Athens, Ohio, it is in Appalachia, in the middle of the hills. It was a big culture shock for a kid like me from the city, but being homesick was not an option for me. During my first month on campus, being around teammates, other student-athletes, and regular students, I quickly noticed cannabis seemed to be a popular substance that many consumed along with a host of other drugs. Cannabis was always the one thing I felt was the perfect balance for me.

However, there was one defining moment that stood out. One of my teammates invited me to a party-themed "Track Meet." There were about twenty or more people in an apartment with about four pounds of cannabis on the kitchen island, and blunt after blunt was being rolled. I soon figured out why it was called a track meet. The blunts kept going in rotation like a track relay race, and when one blunt was finished, another was being rolled and put into rotation.

That day I consumed more cannabis in one sitting than I ever did in my life and had a blast! There was no hangover or feeling of being out of control; I was just really high, which led to the munchies, relaxing, jokes, and great sleep.

Unfortunately, the next day I got the dreaded call from our team trainer that they needed me to come in for a drug test and panic automatically set in. It was such a quick turn of events, and my career flashed before my eyes because, as a big recruit, the last thing I wanted my coaches to discover was that I was a cannabis consumer. After all, my image was very important. I was the clean-cut, private school kid from a two-parent household with not a blemish on my resume.

I decided to hit up the local head shop to get a detox drink, hoping to mask the weed in my system. I went through a workout, practiced, and drank a bunch of acidic drinks to try to sweat as much as possible before I went in for the test. Back then, failing a drug test was a light penalty which meant you might lose a quarter or two of playtime, but thankfully I was redshirting. This meant I was not playing that year, only training and practicing. So the worst-case scenario for me was looking like a stoner to my coaches.

I was nervous because I did not know what the repercussions would be, and from what other players told me, the only way you find out about the test outcomes was if you failed. So throughout the coming weeks, I had nerves just waiting for a call to confirm the worst, but that call never came, and I felt like I had dodged a bullet.

This did not stop me from consuming cannabis though, but I did cut back and consciously made an effort to be more balanced in my consumption.

Fast forward to my redshirt freshman year, I had been around for a year and put on some muscle, so I felt more prepared and ready to compete. In my first collegiate game against UCONN, I managed to get my first career interception, and I would get five more throughout the season, which placed me in the top ten athletes in college football in interceptions and top four freshmen in the nation, ultimately earning me Freshman All-American and All-Conference honors.

As a collegiate athlete, it is a constant grind where you wake up early in the morning to train, lift weights, attend classes, watch films, do physical therapy, have a social life, and do school work. This can be a lot, but I noticed cannabis helped me focus when needed and relax at other times.

As an athlete being able to relax and rest is essential to recovery. Once I noticed cannabis truly helped me manage my intense lifestyle, I was willing to take the chance and consume it consistently. Even if it meant potentially failing a drug test.

During my redshirt sophomore year, hoping to have another breakout year, I was injured in the first quarter and suffered a season-ending injury spraining my left foot.

Although I have always been tough-minded, this was a rough patch for me. I had put so much work into my craft during that off-season, preparing to show the world that my All-American season was not a fluke, but God had other plans. Damaging the bones and ligaments in my midfoot, I was given multiple choices on how to move forward. I could have the bones in my foot fused together, get a screw in the foot, or try letting the foot heal naturally. After two doctors' opinions and observing two other teammates who suffered from the same injury and had surgery, I opted out in hopes my foot would heal itself. Thankfully it did!

That season I was forced to sit on the sidelines and not travel with the team while I rehabbed my foot, and my consumption levels definitely grew because I had more time. Unfortunately, the time meant for healing led to increased stress, depression, and more pain.

It was during this time that I began diving deeper into my major, Healthcare Administration. While focusing on school, I also began to study "heal**THC**are," my journey into cannabis education. I gained insight into the structure and systems within our Western medical system and discovered that cannabis was nowhere to be found in the toolkit of doctors and pharmacists. All the while, tons of college-age kids were binging alcohol and all sorts of dangerous illicit substances, but cannabis was still being labeled as the devil lettuce. At that point, I realized the healthcare institutions were lying to my peers and me.

I also had a front-row seat to how our doctors and trainers medicated us. Athletes often were hurt, having surgery, or dealing with something physical, and pain medicine, numbing shots, and opioids became the norm. I quickly realized that opioids were not an option for me. Opioid use caused drowsiness and stomach upset, and although opioids numbed the pain, they did not help the healing of the injury. I also saw the pills being abused by my teammates, which was disturbing. I would only use them when the pain was unbearable.

During my time in college, I was drug tested by the University and the N.C.A.A. over five times in my five years of undergrad, and thankfully I passed all of them, but there were a few where I was nervous.

After graduating from college, I entered the 2013 National Football League (N.F.L.) draft and was selected to try out for the Oakland Raiders as an undrafted free agent. As a young African American male born into working-class America in the 80s, this was a dream come true. I knew I had made it further than many of my peers and those coming from similar backgrounds. This meant that I had made it even if I did not sign an N.F.L. contract. The tryouts were cutthroat, but I successfully performed really well. Unfortunately, I was informed that I was cut from the team, and it was back to the drawing board.

After a couple of months of training, I ended up hurting my back. Receiving no calls from other N.F.L. teams, I decided to retire from football to pursue my other passions, which were business, coaching, and training youth athletes.

In 2017 my wife and I welcomed our first child, and I continued to do my research and advocacy for cannabis and realized I needed to start using my voice in the fight to legalize cannabis. I knew the war on drugs was really a war on the poor and underserved communities that typically looked like Black and Brown folks. In 2019, I decided to publicly come out as a cannabis patient.

After over a decade plus of being an undercover cannabis consumer, I finally felt confident enough to step out of the cannabis shadows into the light once I received my medical card. I felt like I could finally speak about cannabis and not be judged as harshly because I was an approved patient with a true medical condition recommended by a doctor. As I began my advocacy journey, I realized I had a lot of built-up frustration and anxiety because I had been holding so much in for so long. I felt like I could not be as vulnerable as an athlete and, in general, as an African American male.

As a successful athlete, I was used to the limelight but only as a performer, not an activist or advocate. I had no idea what to expect once I began discussing my cannabis journey. Also, as a husband and father married to a public figure, I knew I had to walk a fine line when talking about my cannabis journey to protect all parties involved. When I first began sharing my story, I decided to create a movement called "Athletes and Cannabis." I knew that most athletes could not talk about their cannabis consumption until post-career, even though many athletes consume while playing. I also grew up with a close friend who was a Major League Baseball(MLB) player who lost his career because of failing drug tests for cannabis. I was driven to create a platform to share my story and the story of others.

Although anxious, I was prepared for public judgment and pushback. I knew the stigma behind cannabis, the stereotypes and the perception. To my surprise, there was less resistance to my message than I expected. However, being in the Ohio M.M.J. program did not make the process easy.

Ohio is conservative, and going public does not mean public consumption. According to Ohio's program, consumption has to be in the comfort of one's home, and there are no public consumption lounges. The illicit market is still alive and flourishing, so my lifestyle became a delicate dance of how to go about moving within the program while also being vocal and disruptive.

I hosted the first "Ohio Black In Cannabis" virtual event, which included different Ohio Cannabis professionals, such as Dr. Bridget Cole Williams, State Representative Juanita Brent, Kevin Greene, Vice-president of the Cleveland School of Cannabis, and others. Ohio does not have a social equity clause in our legislation for ownership, so becoming a licensed cannabis business owner was nearly impossible. I figured working in the ancillary area would be the most cost-effective and impactful way to accomplish my message.

Things became challenging during the pandemic being a stay-at-home father of two toddlers; however, I knew if I created virtual events, I could still make a change. During this time, cannabis businesses became essential services in Ohio. I still did not see as much talk, education, or resources flowing to the average citizens as I liked, so I started another platform called the Ohio Cannabis Report with one of my industry friends and Courage in Cannabis Author in Book One, Broderick Randle II, in hopes of sharing stories, education, and information from Ohio patients and industry insiders. While hosting the "Ohio Cannabis Report" on Instagram, I realized there were so many stories out there, and people just needed a platform to be heard. Our listeners shared that they felt empowered by our movement and inspired by the stories of others.

Today I am excited to say that I took the risk of putting myself and my story out there. Now it has me in conversation with some amazing people doing meaningful work in the cannabis community and hopefully impacting the lives of others positively.

Cannabis has a long history of doing just that. I aim to continue creating opportunities and platforms for these conversations.

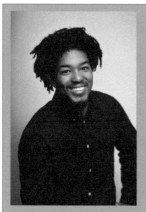

Gerald A. Moore Jr.
President of Green Environmental
Outreach (GEO)
www.geononprofit.org
moore.gerald7@gmail.com
IG: @athletesandcannabis

Learn more about Gerald
at www.courageincannabis.com:

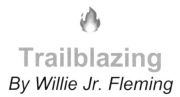

Trailblazing
By Willie Jr. Fleming

In 1997, I remember smoking cannabis in Cabrini Green, the public housing project on the Near North Side of Chicago, Illinois. This was in my early adult years and I used it for social reasons. This would lead to my arrest for possession with intent to deliver.

In 2013, I organized and advocated for medical marijuana to be legalized because the medicine for the pain I was taking was a bit extreme.

In 2019, I organized and advocated for cannabis to be legalized for recreational use so that those like me could have our records expunged in an opportunity to have an ownership interest in this industry.

July 15, 2021, was a day that changed my life forever. I received a call and an email informing me that I would be among the first Blacks in my state to be awarded multiple social equity licenses to own and operate a cannabis facility!

Call it what you want, Legacy to Legal, but remember to call me a pioneer, a trailblazer, and an Equity Enforcer.

WILLIE JR. FLEMING

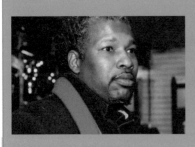

Willie Jr Fleming
ChiCann
FB: Chicannabiz
jr@chicann.com

Learn more about JR Fleming
at www.courageincannabis.com:

Legacy

By Johnnie and Leo Curry

For almost four decades, cannabis has had an immense impact on my life. Despite not smoking it for personal use, it made up the primary source of my livelihood. Cannabis was illegal back then, and being found in possession of it could lead to lengthy incarceration.

My identical twin, Leo and I were intrigued by the notion of striking it big one day, enough to take on the risk that accompanied selling drugs. The financial trappings of success that yield money, power, and respect seemed so compelling for us to embark on this uncharted journey.

For ten years, we trafficked cannabis and cocaine valued at an estimated $200 million and ran one of the largest and most infamous drug operations in Detroit's history. In 1988, we were hit with a federal indictment for carrying out a criminal organization. Our fate was ultimately sealed. The realization that our lives would be forever undone by a mandatory sentence of at least twenty years, with no hope of being released, was etched in our minds.

It was these life-altering circumstances that profoundly shifted our outlook on life. Today, we have overcome all odds and emerged as successful businessmen in the booming cannabis industry.

Here's How it All Began

We grew up during the 60s on the eastside of Detroit, as our family had relocated from Tennessee in search of a better life. We were among the great migration of families that made their way to Detroit—mainly looking for work on the assembly lines at the Henry Ford auto plants.

Their wages, while modest by today's standards, were paying better than most jobs. Unfortunately, factory closings and stagnation in the industry would defer those dreams.

My earliest memory of Detroit was the race riots of 1967, known as the Twelfth Street Riot or Detroit Rebellion. According to some published reports, the police raided an after-hour spot celebrating the welcoming home of two young Black Vietnam soldiers. Mostly, everyone who had gathered to celebrate the homecoming was arrested and charged. Those arrests would spark one of the bloodiest riots in Detroit's history. You could feel the anger and despair in the air.

It was a hard time for Black folks living in Detroit, but it was a reminder that we were fighting for something much greater. The rallying cry for a better life reverberated throughout the city and beyond. The spirit of the civil rights movement was at its peak, and frustration was at its core in the struggle for justice and equality.

Our father, Mack, was a man of few words. He stood six feet tall and had a commanding presence about him. When I was younger, I had to step in a few times when he grew especially aggressive toward our mama. To protect her, I stopped him from hitting her whenever I saw it happening. I did not understand what caused him to become so angry; it was likely over bills that couldn't be paid that added to his frustration. Yet, whatever the underlying issues were, they shattered our family.

Despite his shortcomings, our father was a provider. He never wavered in his responsibility to provide for his family. Taking any job that he could get his hands on, he labored tirelessly for low wages to better our lives. Our dad made every effort to ensure we had all of our basic needs met. However, our wish was that he displayed some compassion for us.

At age sixteen, my world was flipped upside down. Our mama sadly passed away, and it altered the dynamic between my father and me. He moved out, leaving my brothers and me in the house we always knew. My older brother Charles, who at the time had already made a name for himself in the drug business, paved the way and introduced Leo and me to selling weed.

We quickly caught on and began selling it too. Before long, we struck gold by going after heroin and cocaine as well. The profits were enormous compared to what we were getting from selling weed.

Gone were the days of scraping to make ends meet. We prided ourselves on having ample disposable income to give ourselves and our families whatever they wanted. I had two beautiful homes with Olympic size swimming pools and a yacht. You couldn't tell us that we had not arrived. We were sharp as hell. We wore top designer clothing, full-length chinchilla coats accessorized with thousands of dollars worth of jewelry and drove around the eastside in a Cadillac Seville.

While money was no longer an issue, envy, disagreements with other drug dealers about turfs, and possible police interference meant that we had to constantly be on alert and looking over our shoulders. However, the disputes that occurred earlier were ultimately put in the past, and now everyone was unifying to accomplish the same goal—to make money.

Women gravitated toward us like honeybees to a flower, although I had no interest in committing to a relationship. That is until one woman caught my attention named Cathy Volson. She made a lasting impression on me when I spotted her one afternoon at my gas station. Drawn to her beauty, I decided to strike up a conversation. Our connection was strong, and we hit it off immediately. We soon married and shortly thereafter welcomed a baby boy into our lives.

Cathy played an integral role in the success of the organization. As the favorite niece of then-Mayor Coleman A. Young, the first Black Mayor of Detroit, she supplied us with information both from the police and the mayor's office. We were able to outwit the authorities and dodge prosecution for a number of years. In some ways, the police were working for us.

The Calm Before the Storm

Business was still booming for us as millions of dollars poured in monthly. We had several successful business endeavors in our local area, including an event space named "Holiday Hall," a limousine service, a car lot, and two gas stations.

My younger brother introduced me to his then fourteen-year-old friend Rick Wershe Jr., better known as White Boy Rick, a nickname I gave him. The authorities made an arrangement with Rick's family—if he agreed to be an informant for them, his father, an illegal arms dealer and paid informant, would go free and receive a certain amount of money.

For years Rick worked for the police as a source of information until his activities came to an end with his arrest on drug-related charges. Rick spent thirty years in prison in Michigan and later served time for an unrelated offense in Florida.

Rick's information to the FBI eventually brought everything to a screeching halt on April 2, 1987. I was apprehended by the FBI's head of operations, Kenneth Walton Coleman, alongside eighteen other people, including my brother Leo and my friend Wyman. Reality hit me like a ton of bricks. The constant pressure of evading the law was over, and I could accept the magnitude of my wrongdoing. I was exhausted but relieved as I prepared myself to face the consequences. The lesson I quickly learned is there is no amount of money that is worth losing our freedom.

Life After Post-Incarceration

As grandparents today, it's important for Leo and me to establish a legacy for future generations that not only exposes the ugly truth about our past, but also our capacity to persevere, evolve, and develop a better existence that our grandchildren can be proud of.

Since our release from prison, we've been given the opportunity to mentor kids and young adults about the dangers of drug-related activities. Our primary goal is to continue to draw children away from the streets and more into the classrooms.

We want to be able to serve as an example of how not to get involved in illegal drug activity. We are hopeful that our platform will expand to be able to provide support to disadvantaged children in Detroit.

There's been a growing interest from Hollywood executives in placing our life's story on the big screen. We are humbled to finally tell our story and discourage others to not fall for the trappings of street life.

The Cannabis Industry

Despite having an understanding of cannabis, our lack of knowledge of the industry and legal regulations posed a challenge. One of the first things we did was assemble a team that we could trust and one that knew the modern cannabis industry well. An unexpected connection was Dr. Bridget Cole Williams. It turns out we are cousins. Her grandmother was my mother's sister. Because of the dangers of my previous life, we had never met. However, we have been supported and loved by the same family members all of our lives. When she learned of our desire to enter the legal cannabis space, she utilized her knowledge of the Michigan cannabis industry to introduce us to key people that brought us from legacy to legal.

In 2023, we launched Curry Brandz and our first products were a line of flower and pre-rolls called, "Berlina". Berlina was a lavish neo-classic car we purchased in the 1980s at the height of our business. Our neighborhood celebrated it as a symbol of our success and hope that we all could leave poverty behind.

With a growing legal cannabis brand, a movie on the horizon, the opportunity to invest in our community and share our story to help young people avoid the streets, we have truly been blessed with a lifetime of adventures and lessons. The future is bright, and there is no looking back for us.

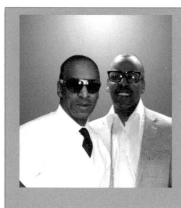

Johnnie and Leo Curry
www.currybrandz.com

Learn more about Johnnie and Leo Curry
at
www.courageincannabis.com:

Weed Mom On A Mission
By Danielle Simone Brand

Like a lot of folks, I used to misunderstand and misjudge cannabis. Laboring under the stoner stereotypes of the D.A.R.E. era, I thought it was for couch-locked and tie-dyed burnouts. I believed cannabis left you spacy, unreliable and smelling of bad incense. I thought weed was weed, and if you used it, you got high. Until I was a mother of two in my mid-thirties, I truly believed there was not much more to it than that.

It turned out I was wrong.

Cannabis is more varied, nuanced, and subtle than I knew. It is a complex matrix of over four hundred compounds, many of which are found in common plants like lemons, pine cones, and black pepper. Of course, getting stoned is possible, but there is a broad spectrum of other effects the plant can offer—from life-saving medical benefits to alcohol-free relaxation and stress relief. As a busy, working mom, I gravitate toward the wellness uses of the plant and find support from cannabis for sleep, pain, stress management, and caring for myself and my family.

Now that I understand cannabis's effects on my unique physiology and can access products to calibrate how I want to feel, I find I am a better partner, mother, and human with this plant in my life.

First, cannabis gave me the gift of good sleep, which is worth its weight in gold if you are a parent of young children. Next, I replaced alcohol with cannabis for socializing and relaxing, and voilà, my chronic migraines subsided. Learning how to dial in my cannabinoids, timing, and dosage helps me channel the more creative and patient mama I strive to be. And cannabis boosts my motivation for self-care—hello, yoga, meditation, and movement!

Cannabis's well-known mood-enhancing benefits are, quite honestly, a game-changer in my life as a parent. When micro-dosing, I get a subtle shift that helps me immerse myself in watercolor projects or backyard games of frisbee with my two kids. With cannabis, I do not morph into a supermom—just a slightly less frazzled version of myself, a mom who can set aside her never-ending to-do list and focus on my children's emotional needs. Cannabis gives me the gift of presence; I use it to tune in, not tune out.

While writing my book, *Weed Mom: The Canna-Curious Woman's Guide to Healthier Relaxation, Happier Parenting, and Chilling T.F. Out* (Ulysses Press, 2020), I interviewed dozens of "canna moms" all over the U.S. about how cannabis boosts their physical health and emotional wellbeing. Some moms feel called to share about medical and wellness uses of the plant, while others feel the sting of judgment—or worse, unjust laws.

The truth is that many moms are finding relief with cannabis in their wellness toolkits, but many of us aren't talking openly about it yet. For women of color in the U.S., there are even greater barriers to access and dialogue because of the long history of race-based discrimination around cannabis. I hope as progress toward the end of federal prohibition continues, and on-the-ground access broadens, *Courage in Cannabis* and *Weed Mom* will help change the conversation and curb the cannabis stigmas for all moms.

Across the U.S., cannabis legalization is progressing rapidly, and attitudes are changing. Current polling shows that eighty-eight percent of Americans support medical cannabis access, and fifty-nine percent favor* legal adult use. So let us end the fear-mongering, misinformation, and worn-out stereotypes.

When consumed responsibly, cannabis is a helpful plant that can enhance a mother's quality of life and ability to parent and partner well. So, here is my call to all the cannamoms and canna-curious moms out there; let us ditch the stigmas, shed the shame, and come out of the green closet. It is time.

*Source: https://www.pewresearch.org/fact-

tank/2022/11/22/americans-overwhelmingly-say-marijuana-should-be-

legal-for-medical-or-recreational-use/

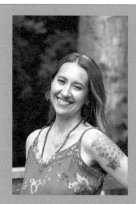

Danielle Simone Brand
Cannabis Journalist and Author
www.daniellesimonebrand.com
IG: @daniellesimonebrand
@weedmombook
Learn more about Danielle
at www.courageincannabis.com:

A Difficult Journey

By Amie Carter

In 2023, the CDC reported that approximately one in thirty-six children in the U.S. are diagnosed with an autism spectrum disorder.

I vividly remember holding my three-year-old son, Jayden, at the end of our driveway while he screamed endlessly as I held his arms and legs. It had become a regular protocol, restraining him so he wouldn't attack me or hurt himself.

On this particular day, as I held him in our driveway, there were on-looking neighbors and cars passing by. I suddenly had a flashback of my baby shower and the day he was born. For a brief moment, I was numb. It was then I realized life with my son would be different than it had been raising my daughter. It was the beginning of accepting the challenges ahead of us, and my heart was breaking.

Just a few months prior, Jayden had been diagnosed with Aspergers, ADHD, and Oppositional Defiant Disorder by two different neurologists.

My name is Amie, and I am a single mother of two. My daughter Alexis is now twenty-three, and my son Jayden is sixteen. Our life has been a whirlwind of twists and turns and nothing at all like I had imagined. It has been a long journey that involved everything from gluten-free diets, support meetings, pharmaceuticals, hospitalizations, and over one hundred encounters with law enforcement.

Our story begins in 2006 when my son was born.

Jayden had colic as a baby and was never content. He cried all the time, to the point that it seemed like he was in extreme pain. He had three seizures before he turned one. I soon noticed he had sensory issues. Jayden was invulnerable to touch or pain. He would headbang. However, he was sensitive to sounds and lights. He would only eat certain foods and rarely slept more than three hours at a time.

At the age of two, when he was at the height of an episode, he was not afraid of anyone or anything. I would have to restrain him often. I would have no choice. It was either that or he was attacking his sister, grandma or anyone or anything around him.

Journal Entry December 5, 2012, Jayden Age: Five

He needs constant supervision and help with everyday tasks. Tonight consisted of him screaming, swearing, kicking, and biting himself, and he threatened to kill all of us. I had to stop Jayden from trying to grab a knife to stab himself. He was saying, "I'm going to kill myself. I'm going to stab myself with a knife. I really am. I'm going to do it. I'm getting a knife, and I'm going to stab myself." We would be at the hospital right now if his sleep meds had not kicked in. For the last three weeks, I have spoken with Jayden's principal at least fifteen times because of his behavior. Today he was sent home early because he was "outta sorts" and didn't like his substitute teacher. The last time he was sent home (two weeks ago), it was because of his behavior again. He was so upset when he came home he pulled his dresser onto himself, and we ended up at the hospital. The time before that, the first time Jayden was sent home, he went by ambulance and was hospitalized for six days. He was only five.

Last week alone, I ended up with a swollen eye for three days, and a separate incident left me with a fat lip. Community mental health comes over a few hours a week, and Jayden is on four medications. Nothing seems to be breaking his pattern or is helping. I will not stop fighting until my son gets the proper treatment. My daughter and I need help. Families that deal with children like this live in an environment comparable to a war zone. We are in survival mode every day. While you can not see my son's disability, understand that it debilitates the whole family.

Journal Entry July 14, 2013, Jayden Age: Six

The other night I was venting. I was talking about how this illness has changed our life dramatically, how my daughter's childhood is unhealthy, and how we are continually verbally and physically abused. I am running out of ideas, solutions, patience and sanity. I was ranting about how much I have changed as a person. I am angry, worn out, mean, mentally and physically drained, and financially wrecked. His needs are greater than I can handle. I am to the point that I cannot even pay for our basic needs; this is too much for one person to take. I had an eviction notice, and our car was repossessed. I have finally hit rock bottom. Who lives like this? There have to be other parents that sit in their car and cry for hours, that have lost their jobs and been pushed to the poverty level, and who live in fear of their child while sleeping at night. I'm getting emotional. Is this it? Is this my life now…? Does it ever get better? Because it hasn't, and after all my efforts in the last four years, this is where I am?

*****

In 2015, when my daughter Alexis was fifteen, and my son Jayden was nine, accusations were made that resulted in Child Protective Services coming to our home.

One night after the kids were asleep, I was seen by a nosey neighbor smoking a joint. I was a medical patient at the time. CPS came to make sure I wasn't medicating him with medical marijuana. I was given twenty-four hours to take my son to get blood work done. No THC was found in his system. They did a thirty-day investigation and found absolutely nothing. While being investigated, I reached out to several people in the cannabis community to talk to them about my situation. I hadn't really considered cannabis for treating my son, but now I was curious.

After learning more about the science of cannabis and meeting Dr. Christian Bogner, who also has a child on the spectrum, I decided that when the investigation was over, I would attempt to get his medical marijuana card. I listened to Dr. Bogner speak at an event. He explained how the brain is inflamed and that cannabinoids (found in cannabis) can reduce inflammation and can allow for new connections to be made. After several days of research, I found Jayden had three of the qualifying conditions that could be treated by medical marijuana.

I set up appointments with two different pediatric cannabis doctors. Three weeks later, he had his card.

I will never forget the first day I gave my son medical cannabis. Jayden was content and happy. He actually seemed comfortable in his skin for the first time. Of course, cannabis is not the only thing that is helping him. We are actively working with several different resources and therapies.

I have observed that cannabis "opened the doors" for learning, growing, and understanding. It put his mind at ease, and he finally seemed comfortable in life. Cannabis helps Jayden in so many ways. It decreases his anxiety, stabilizes his mood, and reduces his aggression. Cannabis has even improved his cognitive impairment. Jayden is testing out at a higher IQ and has developed empathy. Cannabis has enhanced his creativity and made him more self-aware. He even talks about his future, which he never did before. We were able to wean him off the majority of his pharmaceutical medications.

I've learned a lot over the years by volunteering and helping out in my community. We learned firsthand how broken our state's mental health care system is after serving on the board of several non-profit organizations providing resources for families living with autism and mental illness. I helped facilitate support groups and a friendship club and also helped to educate others. I continued my drive by letting my voice be heard in Lansing once cannabis changed our lives.

In 2018, I petitioned the state to add autism as a qualifying condition for medical cannabis. Because of research, previous attempts, and testimony, the state finally agreed to add autism as a qualifying condition. Since then, I have helped several families on their journey with cannabis. It was truly a blessing to our family, and I believe it saved Jayden's life.

Fast forward to now, Jayden just turned sixteen years old and is doing the best he ever has. He is five feet, eight inches in height and weighs one hundred and sixty-five pounds. Jayden has lost all the extra weight he gained as a side effect of taking pharmaceuticals and is in much better physical health. He is attending school, and he loves music, football, cleaning and organizing. I can now have a conversation with him just like I do with my daughter. Life is very different for us in a good way!

I want to be clear, though, this plant is not a cure-all. Cannabis does not make everything just go away. But what it has done is give my son a quality of life and independence he never had.

Cannabis seems to slow down his brain, allowing him to take in information. It seems as if Jayden's brain has made new connections that are allowing him to process the input he can now receive. Since cannabis, Jayden can now utilize the tools he has learned in therapy. He still has the occasional blow-up moment, anxiety, and OCD, although we can now manage it with cannabis.

Cannabis can be manipulated in many ways to manage multiple symptoms. You can alter not only the cannabinoids but also terpenes along with several different methods of ingestion that all have various benefits and powers to truly formulate natural medicine based on what you are trying to treat.

I didn't get a lot of resistance from his pediatrician, which I was surprised by because he really didn't support the use of cannabis. His psychiatrist was also hesitant. I honestly don't know how they truly feel about it, but they have acknowledged his improvements and have never discouraged Jayden's use.

So how do you know if medical cannabis is something to consider for your child? There are currently several different conditions that are approved to access a medical marijuana card in the State of Michigan. If your child has a seizure disorder, cancer, autism, or any other debilitating condition that falls under the approved conditions, you should definitely consider it.

In any case, I always recommend researching as much as possible. And if you are in another state, you'll have to research if your state allows medical cannabis and what steps to take for a pediatric patient.

The last thing I want to touch on is some of the challenges we face as parents who are using medical cannabis for their children.

Once you visit both doctors, you send in the necessary paperwork to the state, and they will issue a medical marijuana card. For anybody under the age of eighteen, their parents or legal guardian will automatically be their caregivers. That means you are responsible for the dosing and also acquiring the medication.

That's where the research becomes so important. It feels out of the norm. We have been conditioned to take our child to the doctor and then to the pharmacy with clear instructions on how to cure the illness. This is similar but also so different.

It takes a while to really understand the science, and it really comes down to the symptoms you are trying to treat. Ingestion method, dosing, cannabinoid additions, terpenes… It's a whole new world. It's also worth learning, and this plant is more remarkable than you have ever imagined.

Give it time. Keep a journal, and don't give up. Sometimes it takes a while to find the right combination, but I can almost guarantee you there is one.

One challenge that I ran into was when my son went to school, there was no way to give him his medicine. I had a teacher call me one time, and she asked, "Can you bring that special medicine up?" I agreed and drove up there.

In order to allow my son access to his medicine during school hours, I personally have to drive it up to him. The law states I park at least one thousand feet away from the school, walk in, sign Jayden out and walk him back to the car. I can then give him his capsule and drive him back to the office and sign him back in.

Not only is this a disruption to the class, but it also singles him out and makes him feel different. It is also an immense inconvenience for the parents as they are not allowed to store it on school grounds.

We are currently working on getting a bill passed into law called "Jayden's Law." We have a committee of three ladies;   Jackie, a fierce advocate in Millington, Michigan, and Maureen, from Illinois, who is the mother of Ashley. She was able to successfully get Ashley's Law passed in 2018.

This bill would allow schools to treat cannabis just like a pharmaceutical. Six other states currently have legislation regarding medical marijuana consumption on school grounds. We have been working on this bill for close to four years. Michigan has had a medical marijuana program since 2008, and I think this law is long overdue.

Journal Entry September 20, 2021, Jayden Age: Fourteen

I started crying after leaving Jayden's school today. I cannot even begin to tell you how proud I am of him. We just had the best conversation about his childhood. He doesn't remember a lot of his childhood. Jayden doesn't know why he acted the way he did and doesn't remember much about anything other than that he didn't really have control. Back then, I didn't know what to do, and all the therapies, medications, and minimal help from the state were not getting us anywhere. There were times I wanted to give up, but I knew I could not. There were times when friends or family would urge me not to necessarily give up but just save myself. It was horrible for a lot of years. And I never thought in a million years I would be where I am today. Not only has cannabis oil saved Jayden's life, but my strong boy has pushed through and persevered through this all. In all honesty, I never dreamed our lives would be as good as they are now. I am so grateful I found cannabis, continued to believe in Jayden and did not give up.

My son Jayden has hit milestones I never thought he would. Don't get me wrong, I always had faith in him, but he has exceeded my expectations by a thousand.

I can't even begin to describe the gratefulness I feel inside. I still can't believe it was a plant that changed our lives.

AMIE CARTER

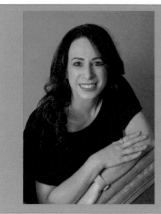

Amie Carter
www.youtube.com/@AmieCarter
www.michiganweedsters.com/
www.jaydenslaw.com/
(https://jaydenslaw.com/)
amie@hearts4autism.org

Learn more about Amie
at www.courageincannabis.com:

Pay Attention
By Christi Chapman

I was raised in Southern California as a Jehovah's Witness, and I had always considered cannabis use to be wrong.

In my high school years, my family relocated to the Pacific Northwest. In my family, there were five of us—an elder brother, two younger sisters, and a younger brother. Sadly, my father was an alcoholic, and my mother decided to stay in a troubled marriage which eventually caused damage to our household. However, with a lot of effort and personal growth, I started to see the positives of our situation. Unfortunately, both my parents have now passed away after long battles with cancer.

In 2012, I made the decision to return to college due to the physical toll my job as a respiratory practitioner was taking on me. Working long shifts in emergency rooms and critical care units in Oregon and Washington had proven to be exhausting for many decades. I had decided to prioritize my well-being and quit my job. However, I found myself unable to participate in activities I once enjoyed, like skiing in Bend, Oregon due to medical reasons.

At the time, I began using cannabis occasionally to alleviate my pain, but it proved to be incompatible with my studying routine. Fortunately, I discovered a cannabis topical that successfully relieved my pain without causing any issues with my studies, and I became a loyal user. However, I was later unable to find the man who had created the effective salve, so I had to take matters into my own hands and learn to make it myself.

Despite having been diagnosed with fibromyalgia and coping as best I could, I now faced difficulties retaining food and liquids. Over the course of eight to nine months, I had lost over one hundred pounds and was overwhelmed with questions such as, "Why was my GI tract affected? What is an autoimmune condition?"

Despite years of working in the medical field, I found myself unsure how to approach my own afflictions. I wondered if cannabis could serve as a viable treatment. I opted for topicals which worked for a while until I became more informed.

In 2014, I walked to the mailbox, which I found to be too arduous, and I happened to meet my neighbor there. I had just barely made it when he remarked, "You're sick like me." After a short conversation, I learned he had Crohn's disease and struggled with eating just like me. To my surprise, he shared that cannabis had been incredibly helpful for his gut and overall well-being.

On that evening, we agreed that I would give his method a try. My neighbor paid me a visit, handed me a cannabis vape pen, and I partook. My complexion perked up as the pink color returned to my cheeks, and the gray, slate-like appearance disappeared. After taking another puff, I felt limber again, which was a stark contrast to my being bedridden for months.

Initially, physicians warned that my prospects were bleak. For instance, one doctor suggested, "Your stomach aches because you're not consuming all your prescribed painkillers. If you did, you wouldn't feel the pain."

However, if the pain subsides, how would he know what to treat?

This was the only thought that crossed my mind. I emphatically replied, "No, thank you!" Always prioritize listening to yourself over others. Our inner voice has the power to guide us if we pay attention.

I began incorporating cannabis into my daily routine, which made a significant difference in my life. After a prolonged period of physical discomfort, I was able to break free from my dependence on opiates.

I am immensely grateful for this positive shift, and I credit Jesus for it. Although I had some previous experience with cannabis during my junior high years, I had set it aside during my career as a respiratory practitioner. Now, however, I see the value of cannabis in my life.

After strenuously pushing myself toward a healthier lifestyle, I am delighted to announce that I have overcome opioid addiction for a remarkable nine years. This accomplishment has taught me the invaluable lesson of persevering for the sake of my well-being.

Sometimes, diseases sneak up on us when we least expect them. However, discovering the healing properties of cannabis changed everything for me. It has revolutionized my life, not just physically but mentally and spiritually as well. To get to this point, I had to ensure that all aspects of my being were nurtured.

It was 2016 In Oregon, I was conferred with the runner-up distinction for my topicals brand. Unlike the side effects caused by the pain relief medicines I was prescribed, cannabis provided a way to alleviate discomfort without lingering feelings of being high. The effect of cannabis was gentler on my body, providing it with more relaxation, and the ability to move freely was a significant advantage.

The human body's ability to produce inflammation is astonishing, but CBD has proven effective in reducing it. I found a need to combine my work as a respiratory practitioner with my knowledge of the plant's medicinal properties. I was searching for ways to administer CBD through metered dose inhalers to asthmatics while I struggled with IBS. Given the importance of clean delivery systems for individuals struggling to breathe, I had confidence in this method. However, after just one month of using CBD inhalers, I gained fifty pounds, a welcomed development that surprised even me after losing so much weight during my illness. When my doctor asked me what had changed, I told him about the CBD inhaler and wanted to share this potentially beneficial product with others.

To achieve the desired outcome, it is necessary to try diverse approaches. Subsequently, the following years were occupied with scrutinizing various products, dosages, and delivery systems. It was during this phase that I discovered my skill for developing formulas. Thus, I began with topicals and now have expanded my focus to include inhalers.

As individuals dealing with chronic illness, it is crucial to embrace stillness in the midst of turmoil. By doing so, we gain clarity and perspective on our condition, which allows us to effectively navigate through its ebbs and flows.

Fibromyalgia is an autoimmune disease. If you have any autoimmune disease process going on, please pay attention! The more cannabinoids of the cannabis plant I used, the better I felt.

I was asked to describe the sensation of relief. It can be described as an energy that I feel, accompanied by a sense of unburdening or lifting of weight from my shoulders, which I once carried. I learned about meditation, but my desire to connect with cannabis felt more interactive and unique. I was unsure of what I was missing with meditation.

Upon engaging in the activity, I had an innate sense that it was beneficial and intended to establish a certain "bond." Through cannabis usage, I was able to establish a re-connection with my inner self. Being brought up in a conservative JW household, the idea of meditative therapy had negative connotations and was considered dangerous. However, I needed to find an ideology that incorporated nature's healing properties and God without getting lost in meaningless metaphors.

Our connection as a human is key to our existence. Our connection to a higher power—Mother Earth—and the soil on which we stand are relevant to the harmony of our own personal journey. My relationship with a higher power is deeply personal to me. Some call it the "Universe," and Others "God." "Yahweh," "Mother Earth," and "Allah" all come full circle back to the same "Creator." A higher power unto whom we answer holds a morality and base for our life values. For me, that is "God."

I've always devoured books like a ravenous diner devours their meal. I seek out literature that can expand my comprehension of human behavior, reactions, language, and the relationship between cause and effect. Furthermore, I dedicate my life to serving others. It is only now that I realize how crucial this service is for our survival.

At some point, I found myself immersed in nature and finally grasped the insight that the Creator had endowed us with—all the natural resources essential for healing and well-being. Along the way, other people offered me advice to turn to plant extracts for solace and recuperation, but this was frowned upon in my own world.

This epiphany marked a significant turning point for me, where God and Mother Earth converged. Initially, I was taught that this alternative method of healing was unlikely to produce a sensation of wellness or completeness.

However, upon deeper reflection, I was left to ponder why this might be so. The concept of meditation was also foreign to me, particularly as society had just emerged from the stigma of substance users who were deemed as lacking in aspiration and ambition.

It was a challenge to reconcile my conscience with the idea that, like all other living organisms, plants and minerals were also gifts from the Creator and inherently intentional in their purpose as medicine.

As we navigate the turbulence that chronic illness brings, it's crucial that we learn to sit still and observe our situation objectively. By doing so, we can better manage our journey and make informed decisions.

Recently, I realized that the most important aspect of this process is the way we approach our thoughts. Engaging in negative behaviors only leads to more conflict and wasted energy. Instead, we should give ourselves space to process and grow, allowing ourselves to embrace the journey and all that it offers.

Today, I choose to focus on healing and finding peace through effective medication with products designed to enhance my experiences. It's been a long journey to find the right balance, but we've arrived at a place where the dosage is key.

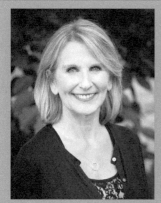

Christine Chapman
www.ChapmanHealthandWellness.com
www.TheBalmb.com
Linkedin: Christine Chapman

Learn more about Christi at:
www.courageincannabis.com:

Excerpt from From

Marijuana Rx The Early Years: Part 1 1975-1980

By Robert C. Randall and Alice O'Leary Randall
(From Chapter 11, "Alone in the Lifeboat")

Available at: <u>The Medical Marijuana Memorabilia Store</u>

****

In this section Robert talks about the time immediately after becoming the only individual in the U.S. with legal access to medical cannabis (November 1976).

"As America's only legal pot smoker I felt like the only man to reach the life-boat. I was the sole exception to a catholic and absolute prohibition. It was a position of great peril and possibility.

The Government sternly advised silence. If you speak, the bureaucrats warned, your small craft could be swamped by other souls seeking salvation. Better to remain still and be safe. It was not unwise advice. I heard unseen others struggling in the waters all round me.

It is a deeply moral question; to be safe and silent while others suffer. But more than   moral motivations occupied my considerations.

The Government promised silence would bring security. But what security is there in silence? Who were we seeking to deceive? If I secretly agreed to the Government's scheme who would I turn to if my access to care was withdrawn? Besides, the bureaucrats would interpret my silence as submission. Most federal officials would be satisfied to intimidate me into muteness. But truly ardent drug warriors would fixate on the danger of my uniqueness. Understanding this threat, such men would not rest until I was erased from the scene.

There is no security in silence. Nor adventure. We were wandering into the last quarter of the first century of the Radio Age. Educated in rhetoric, Fate had conspired to provide me with a unique platform from which to pursue a matter of social merit. Could a lone actor alter the public mind? Would America listen? How might my fellow citizens respond? Six months ago medical marijuana was only men-tioned in the backwaters of the federal bureaucracy. Now it was front page news across the continent.

Having won, why go mum? There were souls to save. Better to trust my fellow citizens and shout into the darkness than rely on a devious Government dedicated to a fraudulent prohibition.

Speaking out, I realized, was a matter of survival. The sooner my uniqueness became typical the safer I would be."

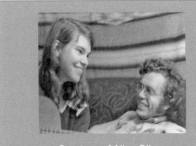

Courtesy of Alice O'Leary Randall

Randall
www.aliceolearyrandall.com
aliceolearyrandall@gmail.com

Learn more about Robert
C. Randall and Alice
O'Leary Randall at

www.courageincannabis.com:

3:33 AM

By Julie Doran

Content Advisory: This chapter will discuss experiences of suicide. Please engage in self-care as you read this chapter.

I turn and look at the clock again. 3:33 AM…

My cannabis journey has been full of ups and downs, to say the least. Through the years, my compassion for the patients and the plant led to my passion for the industry. I've been in the cannabis industry since 2012, but my journey started in 2004. I've been on a long and winding road, and here's how it goes…

I was raised in a small town on a small farm with a big family, one of eight girls and five boys. Coming from a small town, most people knew each other, and I found myself really liking this one particular boy. We started dating when I became "of age," which was sixteen.

When you are that young, love is magical. You could always find Judd and me hanging out after school or on the weekends. We worked at the same restaurants, and with any free time we had, we were *one*. Our romance continued all through high school, and when we reached eighteen, we moved in together. Judd and I were building a life together until the most horrific tragic incident happened.

In my early twenties, my life was flipped upside down. My high-school sweetheart had taken his own life in our apartment. After six years of being together and Judd being the only man I truly cared about, this was devastating. This was and still is the hardest thing I've ever lived through, and I wish for no one to ever have to go through any circumstance like that.

One night I came home to my apartment surrounded by yellow crime tape, an ambulance, and several police cars. Before I could get out of my car, a policewoman asked who I was and directed me to her cruiser. I sat through what seemed to be hours of questioning, testing my skin and clothing for gunpowder and monitoring my vitals. I was immediately a suspect for something and had no idea what it was. Finally, after all the berating and dissecting, they told me what had happened. My boyfriend had been fatally shot in our apartment.

I was in utter shock. Thoughts raced through my head like, did this really happen? Was this actually real? What happened? How'd it happen?

Yes. It was real. Very real.

My heart sank from my chest. It felt like it was falling into the deepest ocean, an endless pit.

It took me staring at a wall for ten days to realize I needed help. Doctors immediately put me on several medications for trauma, PTSD, anxiety and depression.

I didn't like taking pills in the first place, and now they had me taking a handful every day. I couldn't function, none of the pills seemed to work, and on top of it, I suffered from horrible side effects. I couldn't concentrate at work. I couldn't sleep, and if I did manage to get some sleep, I would have horrible nightmares. I couldn't eat. I had no energy to do anything. I was so weak and tired all the time. Of course, I had a big family and many friends, but I never wanted to spend time with them or do anything because I was so numb, both from trauma and pharmaceuticals.

This was when I started leaning on cannabis as my medicine. It was actually the only thing that helped with all the emotional trauma and physical pain I was going through.

I immersed myself in work. I worked two and three jobs, usually working sixty to eighty hours a week and kept myself busy all the time. I didn't have time to *feel* if I remained busy.

However, I started noticing how much better I felt in all ways when I used cannabis, from being able to get myself out of bed to accomplishing major goals at work. I started going out with friends a little more. I would meet up with my family more often. I went back to church (although I've turned more spiritual than religious through my journey). I started to feel a little more *normal* day by day.

I took my last pill a year after that horrible tragedy, knowing the pills never helped me anyway. And yet, I kept my cannabis use somewhat hidden for the next several years. My closest friends and family knew I used it, but it was still so demonized I feared that no one understood how much it medically helped me.

I still use it to this day, but now the world knows. I don't hide it, and I actually go around telling everyone how beneficial it is in almost any situation. I ask them what they're taking medication for, and almost one hundred percent of the time, cannabis would help with the issues they were trying to address with pharmaceuticals. Sometimes pharmaceuticals are needed and life-changing for some, but I would always rather try something natural first.

After years of use, in 2012, I saw the legalization movement start to pick up its pace. That's when I decided to go into the cannabis industry. Still very early and very controversial, no one wanted to hear how cannabis could change people's lives. No one wanted to help me in the industry. My family actually fired me from my job working for them because of how I felt about the plant and how they couldn't jeopardize their business if their customers found out I was involved with "the devil's lettuce." I knew I had some hurdles to jump over, but that was okay. I didn't let that bother me.

3:33 AM… I would often wake up at this time. It was often the only time I would have deep thoughts and ideas and receive direction on what to do. For some reason, I had a burning in my soul.

To recap: I was raised on a farm in a family of thirteen children, so when I said I had some family, I meant I had *some family*. Most of them didn't support this plant and looked down upon everything I was doing. But not my dad. (Don't tell anyone, but I'm Dad's favorite.)

Well, being a farmer and knowing and loving what this plant can do—*change lives*—I went on with my mission. My mission was to keep this medicine safe and clean for its users.

With legalization, the growers from the West Coast emerged with their two to three pounds of flower per plant and, oh, all the stuff they could make their plant do with all the *chemicals* they would feed it.

I made it my mission to create the best organic nutrient line specifically formulated for cannabis. I immersed myself in all the education I could about the plant. (Not much was publicized on the subject yet.) I learned all I could about cultivation, plant needs at certain growing times, different products and techniques—all of it. I spent two years studying cannabis growth and production, carefully tracking what nutrients the plants naturally utilized best and specifically what they needed at different times throughout their growth cycle.

I wanted to create the perfect cannabis fertilizer to ensure the products from the plant would remain clean and organic. And all my research led to the creation of Meigs Fertilizer.

As I learned more about the history and use of the cannabis plant in industry and medicine, I knew it was one of God's greatest creations. No doubt, cannabis products have been used medicinally throughout time and across the globe for a variety of symptoms with much success.

After a couple of years, I naturally learned more about the terpene profiles of different cannabis plant varietals and how different terpenes were improving people's lives in ways I never imagined. Terpenes are produced in tiny, white, hair-like outgrowths that cover cannabis and hemp flower called trichomes. Terpenes give cannabis its different medicinal attributes.

I wanted to produce a product that would help my father, who is a diabetic. He had been on all the usual medications, but still, his diabetes was uncontrolled, and he did not feel well. This led to the creation of my CBD products. After my father started taking CBD, he was shocked that within one week, his blood sugar levels were cut in half. Over the next few months, he continued with CBD products. Despite taking less and less of his other medications, his sugar level remained controlled, and he felt better than he ever had.

Before I planted my first crop and before I could have ever suspected what direction was next in my journey, I had a vision. I saw myself in the clouds in a cannabis field and was told, "This is the earth's medicine." The first time this happened, I was shocked and in tears. I immediately called my mother, who assured me that God has a plan for me and this might be my purpose. That was just one of many visions and encounters to come, and these visions or encounters have propelled my work and love of the plant even further.

Considering that CBD products were more helpful for my father than his pharmaceutical medications, I knew it must be made available to the public and knew Ohio was the perfect place to grow it. But I needed to educate the farm industry and the legislators. This led me to the Ohio Statehouse, and in 2017 and 2018, I met with eighty-nine of our one hundred and thirty-two representatives to educate them regarding the importance of starting a legal hemp program in Ohio and the legalization of cannabis across the state.

To help start the hemp farming industry, I held the first Ohio Hemp (Farm) Summit. That was in 2018. This meeting educated farmers on all aspects of growing the cannabis plant for medicinal and/or industrial use. It also informed cannabis supporters of the legalization efforts we needed to carry out and how they could participate. Many Ohio farmers were excited to be a part of this new *budding* industry which led me to the creation of the Ohio Hemp Farmers Cooperative. Soon after, the 2018 Farm Bill was signed, which legalized hemp and its production on a federal level.

3:33 AM… Again and again. All throughout 2017, 2018 and 2019, I would often find myself waking up at 3:33 AM. In 2019 after one of my summits, I was confronted by a complete stranger who told me, "You often get direct downloads from God in the middle of the night, usually in the forms of lists."

Ah-ha! My lists! That's exactly what I do every time I wake up at 3:33 AM. For some reason, I'm wide awake, so I grab my phone and start making my lists. Half the time, I don't know why I put things on these lists, and sometimes I don't even know whose name I just jotted down, but I always find out later.

I continued my work with the Ohio Hemp Farmers Cooperative to ensure our members were using reliable genetics that produced both safe and effective hemp products. After many meetings, phone calls and emails, hemp was legalized in Ohio.

As soon as I could, I started Trichome Crops Farm and planted my first hemp crop of over four thousand plants. Of course, my dad was out in the hemp field with me every day, tending to the cannabis plants. I can not express how much time, love, and labor it takes to raise these big, beautiful medicinal plants, but it's worth it! Together we are committed to organically growing the best hemp and helping forge the industry into a reality. We are now producing our new "Friends and Family" hemp products, grown and manufactured in Ohio.

What I liked the most was when my salesman called me the "Erin Brockovich of weed." My aim is to help as many people through the stresses in their life in all-natural alternative ways. Freedom feels so good, and I want to help as many people as I can see the light for a better future. Life is a one-time offer, and we need to use it well.

My journey in the cannabis industry continues along with all the cannabis supporters in Ohio and reaching throughout the United States of America. I will continue to fight for legal home growth and adult use. Together we can make that a reality.

The pain of my boyfriend's death is never that far away. People who know me can still see it in my eyes. Maybe 3:33 AM was God guiding me and helping me find positive energy to fulfill my goals.

Through this tragedy, I found cannabis which became my guide toward healing and was the gift I received to help others.

***If you struggle with suicidal thoughts, help is available: 988 Suicide & Crisis Lifeline. Text 988 or chat to 988lifeline.org

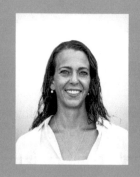

Julie Doran
www.ohiofriendsandfamily.com
jdoran12@att.net

Learn more about Julie
at www.courageincannabis.com:

The Fight of My Life
By Jennifer Isbell Boozer

I was born a fighter. I come from a long line of strong Cajun women who taught me to speak my mind and never back down from a challenge. But even my bold upbringing could not prepare me for the battlefields I would find myself on in life or how significant my faith in God would be in keeping me on my feet.

When I was only twenty-five years old, I had to fight for my life. My son, Elijah, was born brain-dead, my uterus ruptured, and I nearly bled to death. I had to fight for his tiny life for five days, half alive myself, until we made the heart-wrenching and compassionate decision to take him off of life support. I then had to resist the urge to lay in his grave beside him after we said our final goodbyes.

I wrestled with the torment of grief while healing and caring for my living son, Isaiah, who was only two and needed his mother. I had to claw my way through the fear of not having any more children until the miraculous birth of my daughter, Bella. The pain of losing Elijah eventually became a battle for my mind and body when the pain pills, meant to help me cope, became my only comfort. I spent a decade numb to the life happening around me while sinking into a black sadness that eventually twisted into a fascination with my own death.

Once again, in a fight for my very next breath, I warred against the need opiates created in my body and the corrosive thoughts that occupied my every waking moment. But by God…I was delivered from the prison of addiction and redeemed to a worthwhile existence I did not deserve. I have been clean since October 31, 2014.

In November 2017, I was given my greatest weapon: CBD. In one serving, the plant changed my life in profound and vast ways. I was voracious for information about the what, why, and how, and trying to understand why no one seemed to know about this amazing plant medicine. Learning everything I could became a daily quest and started me down the path that would be my life's calling and cause. I saw the need for answers and resources going unmet, and I prayed for the chance to help change it.

Opening a business is hard, no matter who you are. Starting one after seventeen years at home with my children, almost no money, and zero experience, sans a mentor or even someone to emulate. Well, that is my business story. Add to that the extra challenges we face in the cannabis industry with licensing, banking, insurance, marketing obstacles, and more. It feels downright impossible some days. And did I mention I am a woman and live in Alabama? I am often grateful now that I had no idea how difficult this would be because I may have looked before the leap and chickened out!

God gave me the name "CannaBama" and dropped a vision for it in me that is so vast I will not live to see it to full fruition. There was suddenly a fire in my belly that had never existed before CBD. I could not help but find a joy I had never known in doing this work. Helping people turn around awful, hopeless situations. I was helping addicts like myself on top of it all, which gives me great hope each day to keep attacking all the things that stand in my way. I knew instinctively that folks needed a place and a person to go to for answers and compassion—a trusted source of products to buy. No one was doing this in Alabama, so I was eager to try it myself. I prayed every day since day one that it would be self-sustaining so that I could spread the good news of cannabis to my state.

What started as a crazy idea in a two-hundred-square-foot corner of a hair salon has become a history-making, standard-setting staple in my city and throughout my state. It goes well beyond bottles of mystery oil on a shelf and an open sign. We give people what they need most for free and upfront: what it is, what it does, how it works, and how to use it. Education was the catalyst for CannaBama and remains its solid foundation today.

I teach free classes and host a weekly radio show and podcast called "Sweet Home CannaBama" that reaches thousands each episode. I lobby the state legislators for legalization and decriminalization. I host public consumption events and music shows. I sponsor middle school softball and high school basketball to show doubters how harmless the plant is. I spark conversations that impact how people view cannabis and its users.

We were voted Best CBD retailer in Mobile and Baldwin Counties three times and hosted the very first public 420 event in Mobile, by far the largest one in Alabama: 420 Bienville Square. The sky is the limit going into the future for these events, and we still have much ground to cover.

In April 2020, I found myself filing for divorce after twenty years in a toxic marriage, codependent and ill-equipped to face the world alone. I had my clothes, a recliner, trying to afford beds, pots to cook in and towels for the shower. I had no financial support besides my business, which was just beginning to see the devastating consequences of Covid restrictions and a massive loss in sales. It was dark and bleak and had been one of the loneliest times of my life, but I still got out of my bed on the floor and went to work. Why? Because I loved it enough not to let it die with my marriage. I was broken beyond comprehension, and once again, CannaBama saved my life.

I fight on every side, every single day. I was born to fight this particular fight. I know that in my bones. Not one part of it is simple or easy. There are no days off and very few thanks. Nothing is handed to me, and I have to rage for things the average business owner takes for granted. Between eighty-five years of propaganda and the war on drugs, the battle wages on all around for the minds of society. There is much work to do still. I fight fear, loneliness, rejection, and the riggers of single motherhood because the reward is far greater than any obstacle, opposition, or hater I face. Giving people what I know and what I have in cannabis is what gets me out of bed and into my war paint every morning!

If I have learned one thing, it is that I have a depth of perseverance that never seems to run dry and a tenacity I cannot fully comprehend. I have learned that putting people first is always the right move—to value the health and well-being of someone else above the value of a sale. I have learned to pick my battles a little better and not waste my heart on distractions meant to slow me down or even stop me. I have learned to lean on God more than at any other time in my life because I know He will help me see this through.

When life throws a wrench into the mix, and I have to limp along for a while, I know where my strength comes from. I find comfort in those promises. If I could impart any wisdom born from my own experiences, I would say, "Never ever give up on something worth fighting for, especially yourself. And give. Give of yourself, your time, your compassion, and sometimes even your profit margin to those in need." Giving always comes back when you least expect it and in ways you will not see coming.

I am terrible at many things. I have failed miserably at times. But this... This is what God created me to do. This is my kingdom work. I have been called things like crazy, weird, and obsessed, but I prefer names like Cannabinoid Crusader, Warrior of Weed, or CannaBama Queen!

Go big or go home. Fight the good fight.

No weapon formed against me shall prosper. Isaiah 54:17

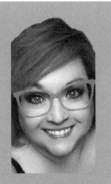

Jennifer Boozer
CannaBama
558 Saint Francis Street
Suite 1A
Mobile, AL 36602
www.cannabama.com
jennifer@cannabama.com
FB: Cannabama
IG: @cannabama

Learn more about Jennifer at www.courageincannabis.com:

"The marijuana laws are based on lies. Everything that governments said about it was the opposite of the truth: *It makes people sick* and actually it is helpful with many medical conditions. *It drives people crazy* and actually it promotes non-violence and introspection… it goes on. To oppose governments on criminal issues one has to be crazy, a fool, a fanatic, or a truth teller. Oh, and courageous. This book is about these people, who helped /are helping to make cannabis legal."

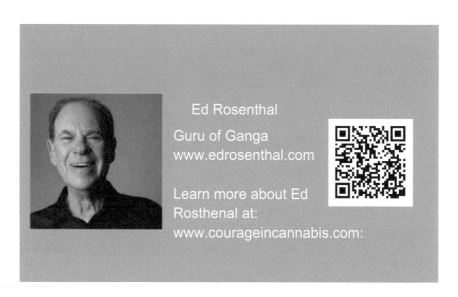

Ed Rosenthal

Guru of Ganga
www.edrosenthal.com

Learn more about Ed Rosthenal at:
www.courageincannabis.com:

Black, Green and Talented
By Axaviar Burrows

I grew up in a family that was largely against the use of cannabis. If they found out you were doing cannabis in any fashion, you might as well have been doing a hard drug. It was highly frowned upon.

Due to the area where I grew up in Canton, Ohio, I was exposed to cannabis in middle school but never tried it until I was about sixteen years old. In my middle school, a large majority of my friend group was either smoking weed or selling it. Since I had always associated it with some sort of negativity, I never had any interest in trying it.

It was not until a New Year's Eve party at my mom's friend's house that I smoked weed for the first time. A few friends from school were associated with my mom's friend, so ironically, I had some of my friends from school to hang out with at this New Year's Eve party. Once all of the adults went to sleep, my friends snuck out back to roll a joint and asked me if I wanted to try it. I hesitated but succumbed to peer pressure like many sixteen-year-olds would do.

"Just take two puffs and see how you feel," they said. I hesitated for a bit, but after seeing how giggly and happy they all were, I got interested in trying it. I took two puffs and held it in as long as I could, then couldn't stop coughing for like five minutes. I instantly regretted it; it fucking sucked. My throat burned, and it felt like my lungs were on fire. I asked, "How do you guys enjoy this shit?"
By the time I got done coughing and drinking a whole bottle of water to try to make my throat stop burning, magically,

everything just began to seem ten times funnier, and everything was hazy. About ten minutes into it, colors seemed brighter, music sounded better, and I had the irresistible urge to eat every snack item in sight. By the end of the night, I was bummed that we were out of weed.

At this point, I finally understood what the hype was about. I was hooked. I loved it. It was the greatest experience of doing nothing I ever had.

After that, I began asking my friends how to get more. I then found out how sketchy drug deals were, but it was the only way to get what you wanted. And that was if the dealer even gave you the amount you paid for. At that age, you didn't know any better, so you were just happy about getting some.

In that era, it was $5 a gram for "mids," which were riddled with sticks and seeds, so you were lucky to get about a blunt and a half's worth. Then it was $10 a gram for "dro," which may have a seed or two and $20 a gram for top shelf, which everybody just called Kush back then. This was around 2010.

I have ADHD, so I can tend to hyper-focus on things I have an interest in and want to learn everything about them. Since I just came across weed and I was smoking a lot of it, I wanted to learn everything about it.

Around this time in 2010, there wasn't much you could Google about weed other than the surface-level few positive things, of course, and the majority of negative things and propaganda that we all know about today.

After a few months of secretly smoking after school and mixed martial arts (MMA) training, one of my younger foster brothers caught me coming home smelling like weed after MMA practice. He was somewhere around thirteen to fifteen years old at that time. His name was Tyler Carter. Tyler grew up a country boy in a rural area of Ohio. Tyler and I were very close, and he started telling me that he remembered his father used to grow cannabis in their barn when he was younger. Tyler also said he remembered a lot of the things his dad did to take care of the plants. At that moment, a lightbulb went off in my head, and I realized with all those seeds I had, "I could grow this shit and save money!"

I had no idea how hard it was to grow cannabis, but I thought I was on to something. At this point, I would pick Tyler's brain for everything he could remember about his father's weed growing. He told me that you need special lights, special dirt, special chemicals, and that it took a lot of time trimming it to make it grow properly. I was impressed at the amount of shit he knew about growing weed, but he was a super smart kid. It was thanks to Tyler that I started to wormhole and research everything I could find on the internet at that time about cannabis cultivation. That was in 2010.

I would spend hours every day after school smoking and researching cannabis, cultivation, and all of the benefits that cannabis had. I even began to try to educate all of my "pothead" friends at the time about the medical benefits of cannabis. I had a fascination-driven obsession with everything cannabis. It was so bad that my friends would say I was ruining the smoke sessions by trying to educate them on various cannabis topics. I would often hear, "Shut up nigga and just smoke the fucking weed," or "Poindexter ass nigga" and then we all would just start laughing.

At this point in time, no one really knew that "weed" had any medical benefits other than making you happy and high. After a while, I became known as the weed expert in school. I was the guy a lot of my friends were getting weed from because they trusted me, and I always had options. I was like a mini dispensary. You had options, and I would tell you the different effects of each. Upper or downer. Did you want to laugh and have energy or be stoned and stuck on the couch? I made sure to have a strain for all occasions.

I also became the guy that a lot of people wanted to get high with for the first time, which I thought was cool. And for all of my friends who wanted to try it for the first time, I would make sure to tell them everything I knew about it before I'd let them try it, like how it could affect them, good and bad, along with whatever cannabis history I had learned at the time. If you knew who I was in high school, you associated me with weed, being high and laid back twenty-four/seven. The majority of my teachers also knew but left me alone because my grades were always on point.

I also had a client that was about seventy to eighty years old that my Grandma Pam, who was a huge cannabis advocate, connected me with. He said it helped him with his arthritis and other pains he had from aging. This was one of the first times I had seen firsthand the medical benefits of cannabis. He said since he started smoking cannabis, he cut back on his addictive pain medications. This led me to further dive into a wormhole on any medical cannabis studies I could come across.

In 2011, at the age of seventeen, it had been about a year since I officially became a "stoner." I found myself not having to take my ADHD medication since starting my cannabis consumption, and I thought I would try my hand at growing since I was spending so much on budgeting and buying weed. Until then, I was selling it just so I could break even to supply my habit, essentially smoking for free and having a few extra dollars to play with.

I took all of Tyler's knowledge and everything I could find on OG Grower, YouTube, and forums. I had my first plant growing in the closet of my room while living with my mom and managed to keep it a secret for a while. Eventually, I got busted by my mom, but that's for another story. I was growing my first plant in a huge old-school popcorn tin that you would find at your grandma's house. In that, I installed a few small CLF coil lights, a milk jug cut in half with some regular potting soil, and Miracle Grow tomato nutrients. I began to grow and kill a bunch of tiny plants. But there was something fulfilling about germinating a seed and watching it grow that just further fueled my fascination for cannabis. Everything in that little container taught me all the fundamentals I needed to learn to go on to run multiple large indoor and outdoor cannabis operations in the future.

In 2011, I was a junior in high school, and at this time, my older brother was taking law classes in college and got an internship at a legal cannabis law firm in Ann Arbor, Michigan. Michigan was one of the only few nearby states that were legal at the time. He took me and a few of his friends on a weekend vacation there, and it opened my eyes to how the legal market was and how accepted it was in society there. It was unfathomable coming from the strict zero-tolerance state of Ohio. I had friends getting in trouble in the legal system by getting pulled over with weed to coming to where they have places called dispensaries where you can openly buy weed and even legally grow it. Michigan even had public weed-smoking events like "Hash Bash" that they were known for.

That was a pivotal moment in my life. It completely changed my way of thinking about the plant. That exposure set me apart from everyone who liked cannabis around me back home. I shared how weed was legal and how I could see the rest of the country following suit soon, and that Ohio would be a legal cannabis state in the future. Everyone thought I was crazy. I was so "crazy" that around this time, I made up my mind that I would work with cannabis in some way for the rest of my life.

Soon after that trip, I took a horticultural elective in high school. In 2012, my senior year, there was a board in the hallway that shared the placement of all seniors that applied for college and the major they were interested in. Teachers and other students in my class thought I was wild for my major of choice being horticultural science or botany. Once they found out my goal, they just thought it was some far-fetched "pothead dream." I would get, "So you just think you can grow weed for a living?" and "Wow, you just want an excuse to smoke forever" from multiple people. But they didn't have the exposure and insight I had from that single trip to Michigan. The majority of people at that time had no idea cannabis was even legal in Michigan or anywhere at that time. So I thank my brother Anthony Burrows Jr. for that single weekend trip. It literally changed the trajectory of my life.

Unfortunately, I didn't get accepted into any of the schools I applied for with botany or horticulture majors. So,

I went to the same college as my brother, but for hospitality management and a minor in culinary arts. This was circa 2014.

Cooking was another passion of mine. While in culinary school, I had a few plants growing in the closet of whatever apartment I was staying in and always stayed up-to-date with most cannabis news, education, and legalization happening over the years. I was happy with doing both passions at once, awaiting my time to somehow take my extensive knowledge of cannabis further.

In 2016, Ohio became a medically legal cannabis state. However, I would not have open dispensaries and cultivation facilities until 2018, so I knew I had to figure out something fast if I wanted to get in on the ground floor. I began coming up with a plan. Around this same time, my stepmother was diagnosed with fibromyalgia and was on a number of pharmaceuticals that gave her multiple side effects, so I began searching for ways to help her with cannabis and oils I would make. I found out it was hard to keep track of what strains and products I was making that worked and didn't work, so I began to keep track of things in a notebook.

Trying to help my stepmother find relief gave me the great idea to create an app that would keep track of what was working and what wasn't so I could better treat her ailments (CxCmobile, App Store).

My thought process was that if I was having this problem, there were many others in the world having this problem as well, and I wanted to help as many people as possible. I then founded my tech company, Collective Convenience, a Delaware C Corp. This was in 2018. I modeled it after researching hundreds of hours of Silicon Valley tech start-ups, including every recorded tech start-up or entrepreneurial college lesson that was on YouTube from universities such as Harvard, MIT, and Yale business schools, as well as dozens of hours of videos from Silicon Valley tech accelerators, such as 500 Startups and Y-Combinator.

During this time, I took my business seriously. I was doing pitch competitions and applying to every tech-driven venture capital firm I could to try to find investment. I got accepted into two tech accelerators, one in New York City and another in Akron, Ohio. I even found one through a *Crain's Business* article. Overall, around that time, cannabis was still considered a risky investment for investors. Since it was new territory, they thought it was high risk, even though I was one of the first apps in this medical cannabis space. I found out that the statistics for a single Black founder to get investment were less than one percent. Nevertheless, I kept trying for years. Still, every meeting ended the same—they thought it was too risky, or that I was too young, or that they only wanted to invest in brick-and-mortar cannabis companies like cultivation facilities and dispensaries.

Throughout this time, I developed every pitch deck and all due diligence paperwork to obtain investments, including full business plans and financial projections. Despite all my hard work, it was just a long, lonely road, and eventually, I had to put it on ice until I obtained more capital to push it further.

By 2022, I had watched similar apps come out after mine, obtain investments and growth, when I knew a few had copied what I originally put out in the tech ecosystem. But that's business for you. When I get enough personal funding or the right investor on board, I have things developed that are essentially the perfect cannabis patient tool.

Simultaneously, while building my cannabis tech company, I dropped out of culinary school in my last semester with two classes remaining to attend a cannabis school. There, I graduated at the top of my class in Cannabis Cultivation. That was in 2018. Before graduating, I was the first person in Ohio to obtain badges to work in a cultivation facility along with a dispensary. The Ohio Board of Pharmacy had to change some of the laws regarding cannabis worker restrictions to make this possible. I found that their wording at the time would've prevented this.

Once I made it into the Ohio cannabis market, I went to work for the start-up of one of the largest cultivators at the time, and a dispensary before the market even opened for the public. At that dispensary, I created the way they talked to patients by directing them to find the right products for relief of whatever alignments they were using cannabis for. I created a reputation from all my years of educating myself and had patients from all over the state travel to talk to me. Later, I went to work for a second dispensary, where I had more personal mentions in Google than any other patient consultant in the state. This was from 2018 to 2020. I became the lead patient consultant at that company location. I envisioned my stepmother in every patient I came in contact with and could always find an answer or solution for any patient.

The strategic move to dive head first into the dispensary sector was so that I could "bootstrap" and push my tech company to patients after launching my mobile app in the Apple App Store (see CxCmobile). I was right in my intuition that many people used notebooks, like my stepmother, to keep track of their product usage to find relief. I would just tell my patients to download my app, created specifically for cannabis patients with the same pain point. That was how I proved my "proof of concept" for my app.

I consulted over two thousand different patients before moving to the Wild West of Oklahoma to start a cannabis cultivation facility with a business partner in 2020. This partner I obtained was a patient of mine at my last dispensary in Ohio. Soon after, I discovered he was shady, but unfortunately, this was not until after I had packed up everything I owned in a U-haul and moved to Oklahoma with no friends or family. Nothing but faith and a dream.

To sum up, my "Wild West of Cannabis" experience in Oklahoma lasted from 2020 to 2022., It was truly wild, and I'll save the extensive details for a different book or story. In any case, by moving to Oklahoma, I made my partner around 1.3 million dollars in my first ninety days, from contracts I helped obtain to taking over three struggling outdoor farmers' multi-acre grow sites. I was solely in charge of creating a team to oversee the rest of the season, then everything from harvest to post-harvest and to distribution. Since my partner was strictly financial, he had zero cannabis knowledge but used my credibility to make deals where he disappeared and left me hanging and never paid the farmers back since everything was on consignment. He essentially robbed us all. Keep in mind this was all within the first ninety days of my move to Oklahoma City.

So now, with little money, I had to make things work out somehow. That got me started as a consultant, where I helped multiple grows across Oklahoma. I even got caught up accidentally working for a cultivation site funded by the cartel. And along my consultant journey, I encountered a lot of other shady business owners and practices. I also got finessed by a cannabis school for ideas that I was cut out of after having multiple meetings. They later essentially launched my idea after cutting me out.

In all, I realized that I have a passion and purpose for wanting to help others, despite how cutthroat the industry is as a whole. Throughout all of my time educating myself and starting multiple business ventures in the space, I realize the knowledge and multiple experiences I've gained in the past decade have made me very valuable to myself and the right people. Not many can say they've literally put their life on the line for their work. And to guarantee that they can do what they say.

All the hardships and positive encounters helped me to realize that I need to step back and focus on building something of my own. I am focusing on further developing and building my tech company that I can utilize to touch multiple areas of the cannabis industry. Just patiently building while waiting on the right connections, partners, and investors.

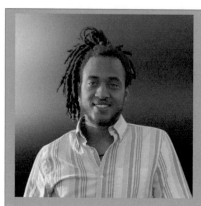

Axaviar Burrows
www.cxcohio.com
axaviarb@gmail.com
IG: @jusscallme_x

Learn more about Axaviar
at ww.courageincannabis.com

Embrace a Life of Mental, Physical, and Spiritual Freedom
By Mary Johnson

At twenty-seven years old, standing five feet four inches tall and weighing two hundred and forty-eight pounds, and despite the stereotypical views about obesity, I felt beautiful, confident and empowered in my skin.

I was an athlete in high school and maintained a slim figure. Things did not change until I left my parents' house after graduating and pursuing a college education while working full-time. However, as I grew older, that is when my weight became an issue.

I didn't want to start experiencing health concerns. I realized it was time for a change in how I approached my eating habits and my overall quality of life. Over the course of a year, I shed one hundred and twenty pounds through sheer tenacity, regular exercise, and reeducating myself on nourishment.

Some people thought I had undergone gastric bypass surgery, bariatric sleeve surgery, or had taken pills to accomplish my weight loss. But no, I did it all on my own. Armed with a newfound sense of wellness and workout routine, I felt called to support my local community in its journey toward better health. To that end, I pursued certification as a chef, herbalist, and vegan, launching two thriving Vitiman Kandie Cafes.

At this point in my journey, CBD had become an integral part of my life. Although it didn't spark my interest initially, my mentor, Chef Linda Berry of Culinary Foundations, introduced me to Cannabidiol (CBD)—a compound found only in cannabis plants—back in 2021 when it was at the forefront of public conversation.

CBD had become a buzzword across the country, and many people were touting its benefits for wellness. However, as an established personal trainer, chef, and bodybuilder, I couldn't afford to risk my reputation by endorsing something that was not legitimate.

While attending cannabis seminars under Linda's guidance to learn how to cook with CBD, I discovered the different strains and types of cannabinoids and their natural ability to heal the body. I realized that CBD had the potential to be a solution for many conditions and was a safer alternative to over-the-counter and pharmaceutical drugs.

I had multiple reasons to offer assistance, not just to my clients. My primary concern was to offer relief to my mom, who suffers from lupus, by easing her pain. I also aimed to alleviate the pain I had been experiencing in my right knee due to prolonged heavy lifting. Additionally, my past weight issues and current rigorous training contributed to an unexpected development of early menopause.

As someone who had reached the age of forty, I found myself struggling with the troublesome symptoms of menopause, such as hot flashes, hormone imbalances and brain fog. It was not something I had expected, and I soon discovered it to be an overwhelming experience. I was filled with fear and sadness, unable to balance my workload due to the effects of insomnia, mood swings, forgetfulness and weight gain. Moreover, I had always dreamed of becoming a mother, but my chances of conceiving naturally were almost nonexistent.

In 2021, after undergoing a series of tests and seeing my doctor, I realized that my only option for having a child was through IVF (in vitro fertilization). Despite this, I decided to put off IVF due to its intensive nature, both physically and mentally, and because of my busy schedule with my business. The only thing that offered me some relief was CBD.

While I may need to consider IVF, surrogacy, or adoption if I still wish to become a mother, I have decided to put my trust in fate, believing that if it is meant to be, God will make it happen. If not, I am prepared to come to terms with that, too.

Despite previous challenges, incorporating CBD into my health routine enabled me to achieve a greater sense of balance in my life. Specifically, I find that taking a 1:1 tincture of CBD and THC, 25 mg each, along with a CBD topical freeze gel of 500 mg for joint pain, has had remarkable effects. I experience improved sleep quality, greater levels of energy and patience, and a reduction in brain fog.

Additionally, the inflammation in my right knee has significantly decreased, allowing me to engage in physical activities without discomfort. As a result of these changes, I have successfully shed 20 pounds over the course of the last four months.

Fortunately, my clients, supporters, and loved ones were accepting of my newfound interest in cannabis and CBD. However, some individuals were apprehensive about trying CBD due to a lack of understanding about its benefits. Rather than recognizing it as a healing tool, they perceive it as a drug. As for me, I can't think of any downsides to using CBD. It's a component of an ancient herb that multiple cultures have relied on for thousands of years.

Conducting proper research and seeking guidance from a licensed and dependable medical professional can be valuable; there's nothing to worry about.

My introduction to Dr. Bridget Cole Williams was a turning point. We collaborated to host seminars that aimed to educate people about the therapeutic effects of the plant. I currently own a line of CBD products under the name Vitiman Kandie CBD. Through my collaboration with Whole Plant, we were able to develop a diverse range of products, including a 1:1 tincture that incorporates both CBD and THC, CBD-infused gummies, vegan capsules fortified with both CBD and sea moss, as well as a full-spectrum CBD sports rub.

Amidst life's trials, I have discovered that challenges are bound to come, but one must never surrender or doubt his/herself. Instead, trust in God, whose grace is sufficient to see you through. With gratitude, I acknowledge that without Him, I am nothing.

Throughout my struggles with weight, a failed marriage, and early menopause, I have drawn from my mother, Loretta Taylor, her strength and determination to persist until I achieve my goals. Thankfully, I have a supportive network of loved ones and trainers who bolster me on my journey.

Today, I am proud to have attained a healthy weight, run my prosperous business, and I found myself again! I am happily engaged to my soulmate. The turnaround is mind-blowing!

In just a few years, I have transformed into a health enthusiast, and I have positively impacted the lives of countless others.

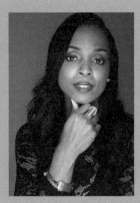

Mary Johnson
Chef, Herbalist, Certified Trainer &
DNA Wellness Programmer
Owner, Founder of Vitiman Kandie
Cafes & Restaurant
www.vitimankandie.com

Learn more about Mary
at www.courageincannabis.com

From A Spark
By Mskindness B. Ramirez, MA Ed

There are those days that seem to have the sole purpose of changing your life in the most profound way. For me, that was March 29th, 2012.

I was twenty-six weeks pregnant with a two-year-old in tow when a puddle in a grocery store found itself in my way. And in the ten-plus years since that moment, the trajectory I've been on has been guided by it.

For several days and weeks after the fall, it was all I could do to get up and shower. And most of those days included severe depression alongside the pain. I tried everything from physical therapy to OTC "safe for pregnancy" meds, even acupuncture and meditation. Nothing seemed to rid me of the excruciating circumstance that had taken control of my body. I was terrified for my unborn child, and I felt like I had failed as a mother before I even had the chance to hold her in my arms.

The fall caused muscular skeletal issues that resulted in a pain no one should endure, let alone while growing another human inside of them. But it was ultimately the system's failure to guide and protect this young mother's healthcare choices that was the *spark* in my decision to use cannabis as medicine and then lend my unforeseeable future to working on behalf of this God-sent plant.

My choice to consume cannabis was fueled by extensive research that I was forced to do for myself, as doctors of the time couldn't or wouldn't discuss it with me. I procured my own plant materials, then made my own medicine, and within days of consistent dosing, I was walking and moving with ninety percent less pain.

We will call the improved mood and uplifted state of mind an additional delightful side effect of the herb. At first, doctors were baffled. But instead of the THC they found in my system being celebrated for its healing properties, it was used to send me down a rabbit hole of intrusive phone calls and glaring side-eyes during my extra scheduled visits. Fortunately for myself, my family and this industry, they picked the wrong Mama Bear to target with their biased and antiquated policies.

It is from this experience my advocacy and my current business were born. Now, I talk, teach and preach about cannabis to anyone who will listen. And all with not one, but two little people in tow.

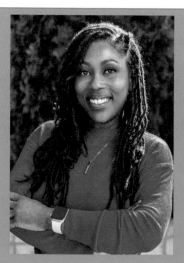

Mskindness B. Ramirez, MA Ed
Holistic Wealth Coach | Author & CEO
www.mskindness.com
me@mskindness.com
linkedin.com/in/mskindness

Learn more about Mskindness
at www.courageincannabis.com:

The Case of the Toking Teacher

By Bronwen Scarberry

Most of us can remember our first experience with cannabis, and I can only tell you what my mom told me. She told me she consumed cannabis throughout her pregnancy with me and continued to do so while she was breastfeeding. She used to laugh and say I was the fattest, happiest baby she had ever met. Happiness was the one thing that weed was guaranteed to bring into our home, and I always welcomed its sweet smell.

When I was fourteen, I consumed cannabis for the first time by swiping a few buds and papers from my mom. That was more than thirty years ago, and I still remember the stickiness and the orange hairs all over it. I ran to the playground and lay down in the grass, looking at the brilliant sky as I toked away. I knew I had found the thing for me. It became my joy and my refuge.

In my late twenties, I let my cannabis use go because of legality issues and turned to substances that were more acceptable and, unfortunately, more addictive. I became the pawn of antidepressants and anxiety medications, and alcohol became my "king."

Alcohol quickly took over my life, and I spent more than a decade drinking pretty heavily, upwards of a half gallon of vodka a day. On June 16, 2017, I checked myself into rehab and have not had a drink of alcohol or a benzo since.

I turned to cannabis again in July 2020 when the orthopedic doctor wanted to refer me to pain management for chronic pain associated with fibromyalgia, polyarticular arthritis, and sacroiliac joint pain. At the time, I had just celebrated three years of sobriety with the help of a twelve-step program, and knew that pain management was not a safe route for me. I chose to get my medical marijuana card because I did not want to return to a life of pharmaceuticals and numbness.

Fast forward to October 2020, when the pandemic was happening all around us. Everywhere you turned, places were looking for workers, and a teacher shortage was predicted. The day was October 20th, and I was getting ready to go to school, not as a student, but as a fourth-grade teacher.

While I was preparing for my day ahead, I knew that I had a chiropractor appointment right after school, an appointment to help me deal with the chronic pain associated with fibromyalgia and arthritis. I put a tiny dab of rosin into a dab pen I had gotten from a local vape shop and threw it in my purse. I truly had every intention of leaving it in my car and using it prior to my adjustment appointment.

However, nothing was normal that day. All of the students were mandated to wear masks, at least those who were attending in person, and students were socially distanced in the classroom. It was very hard to connect with students in masks because of not being able to see their facial expressions.

There were three homerooms, two of which were in person and one was all online, with three general education teachers and a special education teacher rotating classrooms.

To say things were weird is an understatement, and I was mentally and physically exhausted.

The school day progressed as normally as it could, and it was time for me to switch classrooms. My next class was the virtual class, so I loaded all my stuff onto my cart—purse, computer, papers to grade, lunch, coffee cup—you get what I'm saying—and rolled it to my next class.

During that period, I was in an empty classroom. When I removed my computer from the top of my purse, I realized I had not, in fact, left the vape pen in my car. The button for the pen was on the side, and the weight of the computer had pushed it, activating the coil. It smelled like my hash had melted, not a smell that is at all welcome in a fourth-grade classroom.

To say I panicked is the understatement of the century. I clutched my purse tight to my side and went into the bathroom to think and try to problem-solve in a hurry before it was time to be in front of my virtual students. I opened my purse to investigate and realized that I had a mess. I cleaned off the pen as best as I could, sprayed a crap ton of air freshener, and then took my purse out to my car to deal with during my lunch break.

While walking my students to the buses at the end of that school day, I noticed a few different things. First, the bathroom I had gone into had an out-of-order sign on it. Next, the superintendent was standing at the end of my hallway. Then, I saw the union president and a sheriff standing there as well. I didn't think much of it until I walked back to my classroom and found all those people standing there, waiting for me.

I was given a letter telling me that I was being put on paid administrative leave while they investigated the claim that I was smoking marijuana in the school restroom. I was searched by the sheriff and asked to go take a drug test. At that time, I asked if I could speak to my union president, and I told him that I had acquired my medical card in July of that year and knew I would not pass a drug test. I left school to go to my chiropractor appointment, and that was the last day I spent teaching in the classroom.

The consequences, of which there were plenty, sure didn't come quickly. I spoke with an attorney that day, and he advised me to speak to no one except my husband about what had occurred. I went through a drug and alcohol assessment, got drug tested, and was questioned endlessly about my cannabis use. My attorney seemed shocked that I continued to use it.

To make a long story a tad bit shorter, I resigned from my position but maintained my membership with the Ohio Education Association. This allowed me to retain the attorney to continue the fight for my license.

While I waited for the decision about my career, I struggled a lot emotionally. I went through all of the feelings—embarrassment, shame, guilt, anger, and outrage, to name a few—and the choice to resign came partly from embarrassment and mostly to protect my students. I discovered the students were told that I had migraines and wouldn't be back, and I wanted them to think that. At the time, I thought, how could I possibly go public with this? The guilt and shame wrapped around being raised during the War on Drugs ran deep within me.

I tucked myself into a dark hole and an even darker depression. My entire identity was wrapped around being a teacher, and that had been stripped of me. I no longer knew who I was or what I was going to do. I had spent a little over thirteen years teaching fourth grade, and my students were my life. I was faced with the reality that to regain my sanity, I would have to reinvent myself.

Ridiculous laws and controls on cannabis without patient protection language took away my career, and I was not willing to give up cannabis, so I decided to switch gears and join the movement. I started looking at cannabis as a career.

While living through those dark days, I managed to find a position in the kitchen at a local cultivation and processing facility. I spent almost a year and a half working there, gaining knowledge and experience in edibles and in flower packaging. I will be forever grateful for the experiences and knowledge that I gained while working at that facility. The people there really either got the best or the worst version of me. Keep in mind that I was experiencing intensive emotional therapy, menopause, and dealing with my entire identity being stripped from me, and well, I did a lot of personal healing during my time there.

Still, somehow, someway, my personality managed to shine through enough for me to be noticed at the cannabis conference, where I met serial entrepreneur and podcast personality Dustin Kava, who allowed me to share my story on the "because cannabis" podcast, which led to him being my sponsor for this book.

On October 27, 2021, one year and one week after the incident, the state came back with its offer, which went into effect at the end of December 2021. The final finding was possession of medical marijuana pursuant to a prescription, and the terms of the agreement were as follows:

1. Ms. Scarberry's teaching credentials shall be suspended through expiration (June 30, 2024).
2. Ms. Scarberry cannot reapply for a period of three years from the date of execution of the consent agreement. ****If the consent agreement was executed today, then Ms. Scarberry could reapply on October 27, 2024.****
3. Prior to reapplying, Ms. Scarberry must complete the following:
   a) A drug and alcohol assessment with a licensed chemical dependency counselor and follow all recommendations;
   b) A Fitness to Teach Evaluation and follow all recommendations;
   c) Eight hours of professionalism training; and
   d) Complete sixteen to forty hours of community service.

4. Upon re-licensure/re-employment, Ms. Scarberry must complete two years of administrative reporting.

Do I believe I deserved these consequences? Absolutely. I made a mistake. However, if I had taken alcohol, cigarettes, prescription opiates or anxiety medications into school, I firmly believe the consequences would not have been this severe. While I did not receive any criminal charges, I basically ended up with a four-year sentence and two years probation for carrying my medicine. Things like this cannot continue to happen to people quietly, and this is yet another example of why federal legality and patient protection language are so important.

The agreement went into effect on December 31, 2021, which means I will remain suspended until December 31, 2024. I can no longer use the education that I worked so hard for and have to check the box on all professional applications that I had a "professional license suspended or revoked." I went from earning almost $60 thousand annually during my last year of teaching to an annual income of just twenty-four thousand last year.

They may have taken this teacher out of the classroom, but they definitely did not remove the heart and soul of the teacher that lives within me. The God, of my understanding, is an awesome God, and I have known from the very first moment that He had bigger and better things in store for me. I am focused on reinventing my teaching career, but in the cannabis industry.

One day I will stand in a classroom, teaching about the wonders and benefits of this plant to mainstream the utilization and knowledge for others. In ten years (or sooner), I hope people will read this and laugh at how ridiculous the laws were in 2023.

I hope cannabis is seen as a credible medical alternative for former addicts to help them maintain their sobriety while treating pain and anxiety.

I hope my experience of losing my career because of a broken vape pen will be a beacon to protect patient rights and teacher's rights and better testing to determine cannabis intoxication.

I also hope no one ever has to experience anything like I have in the future.

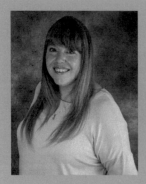

Bronwen Scarberry
bronwenscarberry0@gmail.com
FB: Bronwen Scarberry
IG: @bronwen713
Learn more about Bronwen
at www.courageincannabis.com:

In The Eyes Of A Son
By Jacob Z. Flores

Candy Flores, or as I know her, my mom, has always been the strongest lady I know, not only for being the best mom and raising three children but also for following her dreams and never giving up.

When I was in fifth grade, my mother was diagnosed with undifferentiated connective tissue disease, fibromyalgia and several other autoimmune disorders, which caused her life to take a drastic turn. It affected her ability to work as well as her ability to live her life. As her sickness suddenly darkened her life, she never let it dim the light that kept her striving to fight, which was her kids and other family members.

By the time I was in sixth grade, she had begun to see the light at the end of the tunnel as doctors recommended a morphine pump which would help relieve her pain and give her somewhat of a normal life. Although the morphine pump provided some relief, my mom's widespread pain would never fully go away.

I slowly realized the bigger fight would be the pharmaceuticals themselves. Her long list of medicines, including all sorts of opiates and her morphine pump, did not help my mom. Instead, they would slowly hurt her even more as the body can only take so much before it either stops working or affects the body in worse ways.

By the time I was a senior in high school, my mom had begun to have more flare-ups. Slowly it started to seem like the disease was only at its beginning. Because of complications that happened during her surgical pump revision, my mom ended up going through four more surgeries.

Firsthand, I saw my mom fight the harsh withdrawals of morphine. It is something I would not wish on anybody. It made me feel helpless to see the person I love and look up to go through so much pain.

After a couple of weeks of fighting her body's want for morphine, my mom opened up to the idea of cannabis. I slowly saw happiness and joy return to my mom's life over the years following.

My mom discovered cannabis and its healing abilities. I can honestly say I did not think there was a light at the end of the tunnel, but now I can see there is so much light. As my mom discovered cannabis, she learned not to abuse it and started to do her research. She became more and more knowledgeable about the plant and its benefits.

Over the years, as my mom educated herself, she has continued to be the strong fighter she always was, not only for herself but for others suffering through similar situations. Ultimately, cannabis has not only saved my mom but saved me, too, as I cannot imagine life without my mom.

I thank God I get to see my mom's smile, laughter, and the light she shines on the world. Through cannabis, she is spreading her light and brightening up other people's lives as she educates and advocates to help others live a better quality of life through plant medicine.

Through my mom's battles and hardships with pharmaceuticals, her switch to cannabis has completely turned her life around.

Love your youngest son, Jacob Z. Flores

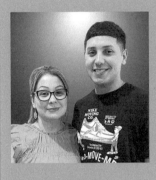

Candy and her son Jacob Flores
Co-Author of Courage in Cannabis Vol.1
canflowercincauthor22@gmail.com
jacobflores99@gmail.com
Instagram: canflo710
LinkedIn: Candy Flores

Learn more about Candy
at www.courageincannabis.com:

The Difference Between Life and Death: Surviving TBI

By Nikki Lawley

***Content Note: This chapter mentions suicidal ideation. Please engage in self-care as you read this chapter.**

My name is Nikki Lawley, and I live in Buffalo, New York. Medical cannabis has been a lifeline for me - without it, I wouldn't be here today. After suffering a head injury caused by a patient, I struggled to find relief until I discovered the benefits of medical cannabis. As a nurse, mother, grandmother, and passionate advocate for medical marijuana, I am grateful for the relief it has brought me.

Often people wonder what nurses do after hours. Well it might be anything from reading books, home health care, getting much needed sleep and others might teach. I was a pediatric nurse during the day and a black jack dealer at night! As a nurse, I found joy in helping people, but as a black jack dealer, I found an outlet for my love of socializing and cards. Customers admired my blend of bubbly cheerfulness, humor and unfiltered personality. Weekends were especially fun as customers would seek me out and I got to know different characters and learn their stories. That was my life before October 11th, 2016.

*****

The Injury

October 11th, 2016, was the day when my life changed forever. I had been working as a pediatric nurse, a job I loved. Helping children was beyond rewarding, and I was proud of my work. The day started out just like any other day for me. I was called in to assist a coworker to administer a routine vaccination to a child, just like I'd done so many times before.

On this day, the fiery 10-year-old boy was panicked and unreasonable after learning about the routine immunization that was to be performed. Despite the parent's attempt to calm the child by offering a special video game for his Xbox, the child refused to cooperate, and all efforts to reason with him were unsuccessful.

The father resorted to holding the child on his lap with the his arms crossed in front of the child's chest. I stood behind the child and reinforced the dad's grasp, holding the child against the parent. This is a standard restraining hold for a combative child. Suddenly, the child tucked his chin and threw his head back into my forehead, snapping my head back against the wall and then back into the child's head for a double impact injury.

I felt completely stunned and surreal at that moment. My adrenaline was skyrocketing, and I couldn't believe what had just taken place. Despite feeling angry and hurt, I managed to control myself and not use any curse words. I raised my voice and scolded the child, "You can't hit adults like that. It's dangerous!"

As my coworker and I were administering the Immunization, a physician from the adjacent room came rushing in and asked, "What was that noise?" In response, my coworker explained that it was Nikki's head. With the doctor's assistance, we were able to complete the immunization for the child. Despite the dad's apology, the child continued to have this disruptive tantrum .

This was a 12-hour workday and this unforeseen incident caused me to run late for my dinner break. I swiftly grabbed something to eat. I received a call from a colleague and shared the details of the event with him. However, while on the call, I started feeling a throbbing pain at the back of my eyes and my skull. My left arm was also numb and tingling, and I began to feel more sensitive than usual to the sunlight. Overall, I could feel something was wrong.

After returning to the office, I immediately felt nauseous. My head was aching, and the dizziness affected my equilibrium. I confided in my colleague that I wasn't feeling right. The staff physician examined me and diagnosed me with a concussion, emphasizing the importance of visiting urgent care immediately. We requested another nurse to take over the remainder of my shift.

Despite receiving a powerful blow, I was surprised to find that there was only minor swelling on my forehead and nose. I was also fortunate that my glasses remained intact. The primary issue following the incident was my heightened sensitivity to light and noise, which caused my head to throb incessantly. Additionally, my eyes felt off, and the pressure in my head continued to increase to an unbearable level. Urgent care provided me with a work note and advised me to take the remainder of the week off.

As a healthcare professional myself, I downplayed my own symptoms and assumed they would improve on their own. I thought a good night's rest would do the trick, but the following morning I found myself unable to move and experiencing tingling, numbness, and throbbing in my left arm. My head was pounding, and I grew increasingly alarmed by an intense headache, the likes of which I had never encountered before. My primary care provider advised me to seek emergency care due to concerns of a potential brain bleed. Unfortunately, I waited for six and a half hours before finally being seen by an ER physician. Despite my concerns, I received no imaging, as he determined it to be a closed head injury.

I felt sick, nauseated and unable to function. I informed my primary doctor of the fact that the ER doctor had not conducted any imaging. My primary was taken aback and sent me for an MRI scan to examine my head and neck. After undergoing the imaging, there was no indication of a brain bleed or any other apparent anomaly. I was astounded. How was it possible to experience so much agony with no apparent cause?

As time went by, my health did not improve, but rather deteriorated even further. I was plagued by a myriad of symptoms that affected various aspects of my well-being, including my thoughts, vision, emotions, and memory. My condition reached a point where I could no longer perform even the simplest tasks and had to rely on my husband to take care of me. My life was spiraling out of control due to my condition, and I had become completely dependent on pharmaceuticals and medical care. The excruciating pain made physical therapy impossible and my repeated visits to the multitude doctors became overwhelming.

I didn't know who I was anymore. I just hurt all the time, I could not think, I could not do anything but cry. I was in a cycle of more and more specialists and appointments and medications, all which did not help. My vision became so affected that I needed to change my prescription eyeglasses five times in just 18 months, and the high-dose steroids prescribed to me caused cataracts to develop. I was a ghost of my former self and forced to take extended leave of absences week after week.

The final diagnosis was that I had suffered significant Traumatic Brain Injury (TBI) and eighteen months after that, it was discovered that I also had cervical instability. That one moment with the combative child changed my life dramatically, leaving me permanently impaired and unable to enjoy the things that had once brought me happiness. I went from being a social butterfly and a respected nurse and black jack dealer to feeling like life was no longer worth living. Gradually, I began to withdraw from those closest to me, and my outlook on life became more and more negative. Nothing seemed to matter to me anymore, and I felt like I was stuck in a never-ending darkness.

*****

Battling The System: Worker's Compensation and Invisible Illness

Even as a nurse, I was ignorant of the complexities involved in navigating the healthcare system, particularly for patients with brain injuries. My primary focus was always to provide care to those who required it the most, and I used to think that the path to recovery was a straightforward process of visiting a nearby hospital or medical center.

But I was wrong.

Securing a diagnosis and receiving proper treatment for my TBI proved to be a daunting task. Despite my knowledge in the field, I found myself stripped of my professional identity and instead became a woman with invisible injuries, forced to contend with medical practitioners who doubted my illness.

Since the injury was work-related, I found myself stuck in a tangle between my private insurance company and New York state's workers' compensation. The insurance provider refused to cover any treatment expenses, while workers' compensation imposed several limitations on the coverage. New York state's initial settlement offer amounted to a meager sum which was outright degrading, barely equating to a year's earnings as a nurse. With no other options, I was forced to claim disability, and that was the end of my career.

I was put on over fifty different prescription drugs by doctors, even though most of them weren't intended for head injury. Unfortunately, the medications came with side effects that were often worse than my actual injury, such as severe shaking, vomiting, and dizziness. Whenever I brought up my concerns, the response was to prescribe more pills, leaving me feeling helpless. Unfortunately, no alternative therapies were ever suggested or considered.

To make matters worse, medical professionals started to question if my symptoms were real. The abrupt transition from being a productive member of the healthcare team to being labeled as a malingerer and fake was extremely heartbreaking. It was difficult for me to fathom that healthcare providers would doubt my intentions or the severity of my injury.

It felt as though I couldn't win. I genuinely believed that if you got hurt, the healthcare system would be there to ease your suffering. At this point, I was utterly despondent. The thought of ending my life entered my mind. Fortunately, a glimmer of hope awaited me in a place I least expected.

*****

The Turning Point

In January 2017, my husband attempted to cheer me up by taking me on vacation to Las Vegas. It was a place I had adored in my previous life, spending hours playing cards and slots and laughing with tourists and locals alike.

But this time was different.

The trip to Vegas four months after my injury was so overwhelming, and I could not function. All I could think about was the pain, how my life was over, how I was a burden to my family and how I was not getting better! The pain was so severe in my head I could not think about anything and I was miserable. I was in a very, very dark place mentally, unable to leave my hotel room. By the third day of our trip, I considered jumping from our balcony. As I peered out at the vast Las Vegas strip alone, contemplating my death, a mobile billboard drove past. It said: "Get your Medical Marijuana Card Today in Nevada."

I had never considered marijuana medicinal - the war on drugs and Nancy Reagan telling us to "just say no," and the vision of the frying pan with the egg - your brain on drugs - were always my initial thoughts. But then the billboard passed again. Suddenly, my husband emerged.

"I can get my medical weed card in Nevada," I said sarcastically. I was surprised when he responded, "let's go."

We decided to take a chance. The billboard seemed to be a clear sign that I should disregard my intuition. Since we had already tried everything else, this was all we had left. I stepped out of my hotel room for the first time during the trip - little did I know that it would turn out to be the journey that rescued me.

On our quest for a medical cannabis card, my husband and I headed to an establishment offering the service. During this time, only medical cannabis was allowed in Nevada. Given my persistent pain, I was eligible for the card, and we wasted no time in visiting a nearby dispensary.

The dispensary visit turned out to be one of the most intense situations I had ever encountered, as the sheer number of product alternatives, categories, and forms of consumption overwhelmed all my senses, aggravating my brain. I ended up taking an extensive haul back to the hotel: gummies, suckers, tinctures, pills, and even two joints.

When I first tried the cannabis products, I didn't have a big shift in perspective, but I did notice a difference. After a day and a half, I found myself functioning slightly better, and I regained a portion of my former self. While my headache persisted, it wasn't overpowering. It was the first time in several months that I felt optimistic.

Upon arriving back home in New York, I hoped to relive the positive encounter I had experienced in Vegas. Sadly, my aspirations were quickly dashed due to the lack of product availability for my needs. Even though medical cannabis was an option in New York, unfortunately, chronic pain was not yet a qualifying condition (it was not until 2018). Even if I had been eligible for medical marijuana, I would have been disappointed by the restricted selections at dispensaries.

After having had a taste of happiness, it all came crashing down again. My despair and hopelessness returned, and I wondered if I would ever find relief again.

*****

A Medical Cannabis Refugee

Having worked at a local Niagara Falls, NY, casino for seven years, I developed many relationships with people from across the border in Ontario, Canada. One day in late 2017, I was texting with a friend in Canada who had been trying in vain to encourage me to cross the border. "We have pot here - why don't I get my medical card, and you can come here and stay for a few days and see if it helps?" she suggested. I took the offer and made my way up north.

I can honestly say those trips to Canada and learning about cannabis as medicine changed the trajectory of my life as I knew it. I became a medical cannabis refugee in Canada. I would suffer for days back home in New York, unable to access my medicine. Then, I would travel north two to four times a month, where I actually improved my quality of life. I found hope again. I was able to function!

Cannabis allowed me to communicate with others; the pain was manageable. Instead of being depressed thinking about all the things I could no longer do and being anxious and worrying about the future and what would happen, I could live in the moment and appreciate my surroundings in the present.

The memory of my fourth visit is etched in my mind forever. Engrossed in a game of Scrabble™ with my friend, I couldn't believe how far I had come since struggling with the same task just a few months ago. Suddenly, the ring of my phone interrupted us, and I saw that it was my husband on the line. A few minutes into our conversation, he abruptly asked, "What's wrong with you?" I was taken aback by his question and replied, "What do you mean?" His response surprised me even more as he exclaimed, "You sound normal!"

I began to investigate the different products available in Canada but didn't really understand why certain products affected me differently and why. I accidentally discovered a journaling app with all the Canadian product COAs - Certificate of Analysis cannabis test reports about the chemical composition of the plant - in a database per brand and product.

Using the app, I generated a personalized report detailing which products had proven effective for my symptoms, as well as for a community of people facing similar issues. With a particular focus on managing my chronic pain, cognitive function, anxiety, and depression, I carefully documented the various remedies I experimented with and tracked their impact on my well-being. Through this process, I embarked on a journey of discovery and learning about the medicinal benefits of cannabis.

■■

Becoming an Advocate: Finding My New Destiny

Canadian cannabis culture became my new obsession. I did everything I could to learn from experts in the field and began attending cannabis industry conferences and events. Newly confident, I began to voice my opinion at worker's compensation doctor appointments back home. Instead of exploring why I was having success, they wrote in my file that I was "drug seeking." My doctors believed that I must be looking to get high because I smoked cannabis, and it wasn't medicine if it had THC. The nerve!

As I gained more knowledge about the plant and its impact on my health, I sought answers through frequent inquiries. From conversing with nurses and medical experts to discussing medical cannabis and sharing my personal experiences, I zealously sought to understand more about the plant's potential benefits for symptom management. Despite my best efforts, most professionals seemed unaware of my newfound knowledge and remained uninterested or dismissive of my enthusiasm. However, after losing my career as a nurse, I felt lost for a long time. But now, by spreading awareness about the therapeutic properties of plant medicine, I found a new lease on life. Guiding my medical colleagues and the general public on this path became my passion and my calling.

Since I first discovered plant medicine, I have achieved things I never dreamed of. I have spoken at conferences, appeared on podcasts, and wrote about my story—all things that would not have been possible without cannabis. I am proud to serve on the advisory board for CannabisBPO and I am also a member of the Americans for Safe Access NYS Patient Advisory Board. These roles give me purpose and allow me to impact the community I hold so dear to me.

I share my story and help remove the stigma and normalize the conversation. My social media following is incredible, and I have been humbled by the support and engagement of people worldwide.

As an advocate, my primary messages are centered on the importance of not judging what one does not comprehend. When it comes to invisible illnesses, it's essential to acknowledge that just because they cannot be seen, it does not negate their existence. Patients are the ultimate authorities in their health management, and their contributions and personal experiences are invaluable in improving medical cannabis research and development. While I acknowledge that cannabis is not a panacea, for me, it is a vital tool in managing depression, anxiety, chronic pain and cognitive function, allowing me to thrive.

Most importantly, I want people like me to know there are options. The medical community does not know enough about cannabis yet, but the information is out there. Cannabis connects my dots, and if it can save my life, I know it can save others.

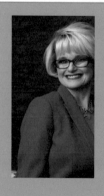

Nikki Lawley
www.nikkiandtheplant.org
nikkilawley1@gmail.com
Linkedin: Nikki Lawley
FB:facebook.com/nikkiandtheplant/
IG: @nikkiandtheplant

Learn more about Nikki
at www.courageincannabis.com:

One Thing Led To Another
By Mary Lynn Mathre

After receiving my Bachelor of Science degree in nursing in 1975, I served in the US Navy Nurse Corps for four more years, got married in 1980, and went to grad school in 1984-85. I had been a medical-surgical nurse for those years, and the War on Drugs was in full swing.

Since marijuana was the most used illicit drug at the time, I decided to do my thesis on the Disclosure of Marijuana Use to Health Care Professionals. However, in my practice, it was not routine to ask patients about marijuana use, and I wondered if people were being asked by their healthcare providers and if they would admit to using it. (Mathre, 1985)

At the time of Just Say No, I contacted the National Organization for the Reform of Marijuana Laws (NORML) to request that my survey be included in their bimonthly newsletter, "The Leaflet." Keep in mind that this was before the internet and cell phones.

I received over nine hundred responses and learned that most were never asked about their use of marijuana, but over half said they would admit to using it because they thought it was important for their healthcare provider to know.

The last question was an eye-opener for me. I asked about their health concerns related to their marijuana use and gave them a list of potential concerns (addiction, heart, lungs, pregnancy, etc.) and "other" as choices.

To my surprise, several checked the "other" box and stated they used it to help with multiple sclerosis, glaucoma, morning sickness when pregnant, spinal cord injury, and more. I knew about its historical use to combat chemo-induced nausea and vomiting, but the other uses were new.

The results of my thesis led me to research the medical use of marijuana, and I learned a lot about *cannabis*, the proper name for the plant.

Upon graduation, I accepted a faculty position at the University of Virginia School of Nursing and accepted a volunteer position as the Director of Marijuana and Health under NORML. Through this group, I met cannabis icons such as Lester Grinspoon, Norman Zinberg, Andrew Weil, and Melanie Dreher, as well as the first five patients in the Compassionate Investigational New Drug (IND) program in which they received cannabis from the US government that was grown at the University of Mississippi.

The fact that our government was providing free cannabis to patients through a little-known application process while at the same time keeping the plant in the Schedule I or forbidden category of drugs was unethical and hypocritical, in my view.

My husband and I were appointed to the NORML Board of Directors in 1988, but by the early 1990s, it became apparent that healthcare professionals were too intimidated by the Schedule I status of cannabis to support its use by patients, and they would never attend a NORML conference to learn more.

So, in 1995, we formed Patients Out of Time (POT) with the goal of providing accredited conferences on the therapeutic use of cannabis. We thought that if we could demonstrate the safety and efficacy of cannabis, healthcare providers would recognize its value and help end the prohibition of this plant.

It took five years to find an institution that would provide continuing education credits for our conference, and so in 2000, we held *The First National Clinical Conference on Cannabis Therapeutics* in Iowa City, Iowa, with accreditation from the University of Iowa's Colleges of Medicine and Nursing. Initially, the conferences were biennial but increased to annual by 2015 due to the massive increase in research caused by the emerging science of the newly discovered endogenous cannabinoid system (ECS).

The majority of states now recognize cannabis as medicine, so our focus on POT is changing to educating patients and eliminating roadblocks to this medicine.

Together with other cannabis clinicians, in 2020, we formed a new 501c3 under the name The Academy of Cannabis Education (ACE). That will continue with POT's conference series and focus on the education of healthcare providers regarding the evolving science of the ECS and cannabis therapeutics.

I also learned of the nutritional value of hemp seeds and hemp seed oil and the environmental benefits of the plant and products made by it.

We have made progress over the years, but the fight will not be over until cannabis is completely de-scheduled and our global leaders begin providing incentives rather than roadblocks to the growing of cannabis/hemp for the health of our citizens, creatures, and the planet.

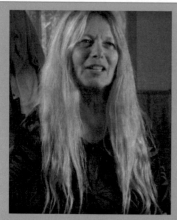

Mary Lynn Mathre
President and Co-founder of Patients Out of Time
www.patientsoutoftime.com
www.acecannabiseducation.com
info@patientsoutof time.com

Learn more about Mary Lynn Mathre at
www.courageincannabis.com:

The Perception Of Cannabis Use

By Dr. Nurse Nique, DNP

"Maybe there is something I need to learn. Maybe there is someone I need to touch."

*****

April 8, 2013, my Facebook post for the day reads, *"Boston bound tomorrow. Another lump, but it's gotta be scar tissue or a cyst because it's where they removed the sentinel node, and it sits on a scar. The mind can make you crazy. So, off to Jamaica Plains in the a.m., then to the gym by sundown."*

It was April 2013, and I called the doctor's office requesting my biopsy results. The woman who answered the phone briefly put me on hold, and when she returned, she responded, "The doctor will call you back."

This was when I realized it was back. This was when I realized my chart doesn't say "nurse." This was when I was, once again, *on the other side of the nurses' station*, and I knew what the doctor was going to tell me. Life experiences, both personal and professional, helped me understand the outcome of that phone call.

Why me?

"Your cancer is back." Those words triggered the anxiety and flashback of the day spent in the surgical suite at Brigham Women's Hospital. It was the day after the Boston Marathon Bombing, April 16, 2013. My perception of battling breast cancer changed that day when I was surrounded by the atrocity that injured over two hundred and sixty people and killed three.

I was greeted at the entrance of the hospital by a S.W.A.T. team and their M-16s opening the door for me as I entered the building. Although my military training in the United States Marine Corps prepared me for war, never did I anticipate I would be stepping into two completely different war zones as I entered through those hospital doors. The first battle was fighting for my life. The other was the immediate threat to homeland security.

The same-day surgery suite had a distinct vibe and a solemnness that lingered through the air and embodied the staff. Suddenly my breast cancer wasn't so serious anymore.

As I prepared to leave, there was another bomb scare. I couldn't do anything. All I could do was wait and wonder what all this meant. I just needed to go home to process everything I had just endured emotionally, physically, mentally, and spiritually.

In April 2013, I was living in Narragansett, Rhode Island, across from the beach. I have a tendency to place myself near the ocean as I feel it keeps me closer to my dad, as he was an avid sports fisherman.

When I got off the phone with someone at the Dana Faber Cancer Institute, I walked over to the ocean and sat on a bench staring at the water, listening to the sounds, smelling the salt water and missing my dad. As the tears rolled down my cheeks, I looked up to the sky and asked, "Dad, why is my life so hard. Why do I keep struggling? What else do I need to learn? Who do I have to touch?"

I sat there, and I cried. I cried with such intensity.

I missed my dad. He always tried to carry me through. He knew I struggled emotionally. So now, with him gone, what was I to do?

I cannot recall the exact timing, but it wasn't long after that meltdown I started a blog on Facebook called "Breast Cancer and Me." I would post pictures of myself and my journey, and I blogged from the bottom of my heart.

There was a sort of catharsis in this form of writing. It gave me the confidence to write to an international audience connected by social media without worrying about what I looked like as I sat behind a screen. I was just someone's perception of who they wanted me to be. I didn't have to worry about "real-time" images or perceived inadequacies from those who wanted to read my words or others who chose to scroll past.

That is how I found my followers. That is how I found cannabis.

I was working as the Director of Nursing Operations in an assisted living community as I started to prepare for my breast cancer treatments. Just eighteen months before the left total mastectomy was supposed to have saved my life, the Oncotype test gave me a sixteen percent chance that my breast cancer would return. Eighteen months later, it returned with a vengeance, and I started my journey with chemotherapy and radiation.

I was so confused, and at the time, had no true understanding of mind, body and spirit wellness. Until then, I had spent the majority of my life wanting to die, and now I was fighting to live. I soon came to understand this to be known as the duality of perception. That is when I began to understand the power of the mind and the ability to shift and change our perception positively, although it wasn't until I embarked on this journey of integrative medicine that I began to understand exactly what was happening to me.

It was in my writing that I was told of the medicinal benefits of cannabis, and when I found I was allergic to the antiemetics to alleviate some of the side effects from the chemotherapy, I began to learn more about this powerful plant.

I reached out to those who appeared to have the knowledge I sought and inquired about the steps to obtaining my medical cannabis card. I applied to the Rhode Island medical cannabis program in 2013 and received my patient card, as cancer was a qualifying condition.

Now what do I do? I thought about this deeply as I also held a Rhode Island Nursing License and was in fear of losing all I had worked so hard for.

I started attending conferences. My first conference was in 2015, Patients Out of Time, and I met so many incredible people, from patients to doctors, teachers, parents, and nurses, to name a few.

I began working in a medical dispensary in Rhode Island, learning more about the plant and the industry, and I did everything from trimming and packaging flower, to visiting assisted living communities and veterans organizations to provide education and bring awareness to plant medicine.

I began fighting for the rights of nurses to use cannabis as medicine by testing positive for THC. I couldn't get a job, but unlike my friend Shondra, I did not lose my license. Was it because I was white?

With what felt like a paycheck away from being homeless, I had one last request from my family; "Please help me get to California. I promise I'll never ask you for anything again."

By January 2017, I had acquired my own nursing position as a home health nurse in Ocean Side, California. I had a beautiful studio apartment by the beach, and I met Nature Nurse at a Woman Grow's Christmas Party in San Diego, California. Her angelic, kind spirit just lit up the room. From the first time I met her, I was awestruck. Over three thousand miles from home, I finally began to believe in Santa Claus again.

The hug I received that night was one of the loneliest times of my life, and it gave me hope. At that moment, she whispered in my ear, "I've been looking for you, Nurse Nique." This greatness of an internal vibration just took over me. I whispered to myself as I walked away, "Nature Nurse was looking for me?" And that day changed my life as I once knew it.

I studied with Nature Nurse through her concept of Post Traumatic Growth utilizing the Lotus Theory that she had developed and her cannabis products that saved my life and my spirit.

Until then, I had never looked at another perception of my life, only comparisons of my life. Shortly after this epiphany to plant medicine, I realized: Nursing taught me how to treat. Cannabis taught me how to heal.

Fast forward ten years later to 2023, and on May 18, 2023 I received my Doctorate in Nursing at Salve Regina University, Newport, Rhode Island. Over those ten years, among other accomplishments, I developed a tool to diagnose Cannabis Use Disorder by separating appropriate and inappropriate use. In 2016, I developed the Cannabis Nurse Navigator position while a young entrepreneur in Entrepreneurs For All South Coast. In 2017, I became a founding member of the Cannabis Nurses Network. In 2020, I received my Medical Cannabis Certification from Oriental Pacific College, San Diego, California, and I am currently a Research Nurse at Olin Neuropsychiatry Research Center doing THC and CBD studies with human subjects as the substitute investigator under the direction of Dr. Godfrey Pearlson.

I have learned about the importance of having a balanced endocannabinoid system through my cannabis use, as my breast cancer is now in remission. I have learned how to microdose to help with my mental wellness. Through all this, I have lived a life filled with significant anxiety and depression, as well as chronic suicidality.

Cannabis balances my mental health and has allowed me to do more and be more than I ever thought possible. I also ignite the endocannabinoid system through music therapy, exercise, cupping, yoga, equine therapy, pet therapy, reiki, acupuncture, float deprivation therapy, light therapy, and so much more.

Struggling with mental health issues for over four decades has left me dumbfounded at the traditional medical system as well as the psychiatric system and why they allowed me and so many others to suffer for so very long.

I will continue on my wellness journey, especially within my mind, until I die, but cannabis has opened a beautiful world of self-awareness and healing that has pushed me past my insecurities and allowed me the courage to positively change my perception of myself.

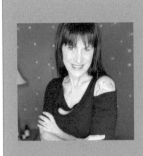
Dr. Nique Pichette, DNP
www.positivelyprocessingperception.com
nique@niqueit.com
Linkedin: Dr. Nique Pichette, DNP

Learn more about Dr. Nique
at www.courageincannabis.com:

Guided By Faith

By Natacha Andrews, Esq

In the world of cannabis, everyone has a why. No matter how many people you ask, you'll continue to be surprised at how each of us came to our belief about the plant. Regardless of how similar someone else's story seems, like fingerprints, no two are exactly the same. I have heard people describe their experiences with cannabis as everything from enlightening to cathartic, alluring, disassociative, healing, destructive and liberating. For me, cannabis is all those things and more. My personal journey is not just about the plant itself, but rather about the historical and social statements cannabis evolution makes about both the world I grew up in, and the one I hope to leave behind.

I marvel almost daily to find myself standing on this side of a debate about cannabis legalization. Among the many challenges of this bizarre journey navigating the murky waters of the movement, has been realizing that despite my current position on things, there is no time-out or reset button in parenting. As I brace myself daily for the sometimes daunting work of advocacy, I know that for my five children, my new perspective is at the very least "complicated." It is that complex tapestry that keeps me humble enough to recognize that I don't begin to know it all, while keeping me hungry enough not to become complacent at the distraction of small victories. It is the driver that reminds me that I should always lead by example and that my audience of five is watching quite carefully.

My children grew up hearing an almost opposite message from me than the one they hear today. The art of balancing who I've tried to raise them to be with making it clear that my activism is in no way permission is an ongoing struggle. One which I continue to rely on God to handle since I have no rational explanation other than that *He* put me on this path, to begin with.

For the first forty-something years of my life, I was what most would consider rather conservative about drugs. I grew up in the "just say no," "this is your brain on," and "crack is whack" days of Nancy and Ronald's war. I not only grew up in it, I believed wholeheartedly every word. So much so that I became an ambassador for the Drug Abuse Resistance Education program (D.A.R.E.) in high school, where I helped disseminate a mixture of truths and untruths to my peers. I carried on completely unaware that the message of morals, values, safety and wisdom I was promoting was ripe with propaganda, driven by an agenda much more sinister than my then seventeen-year-old mind could conceive.

The child of immigrants, I was raised to be unquestioning of adults. A value I in turn instilled in my own children. The choice to maintain that cultural tradition would keep me in the dark for nearly thirty more years before a fated business trip and personal crisis opened my eyes to the reality that my unquestioning beliefs had been placed in the wrong people for far too long.

I began my career unsure of where it would take me, but always with an eye on justice. I eventually became an immigration lawyer, to help families like my own, who's roots began somewhere else on the planet. A decade later, facing the career challenges caused by a wildly unorthodox presidential administration, I decided to take inventory and contemplate what would be next. Not surprisingly, cannabis was nowhere on my radar. I had spent an entire lifetime avoiding the plant and any other thing that might move me away from my perceived goals. But as fate often does, and in a series of unforeseen plot twists, I began to find myself in situations that would challenge everything I thought I knew. I started reevaluating my beliefs about what we call illegal drugs and to shatter my own outlook on plants as medicine.

The first of these fateful situations came 1n 2019, when I took a trip to Seattle. Not only had I never been to Washington state before, I had never been in any fully legal market. What I heard, smelled and saw left a lasting impression on me. I returned from Seattle with a sense of wonder, a newly piqued interest and a gut wrenching confusion regarding how to reconcile what I had just witnessed in the Northwestern most part of the country with the realities of life back at home where the plights of criminal justice and family separation went largely unnoticed by those fortunate enough not to have to worry about either.

It was during this inward search that I began unraveling the tangle of misinformation that had gone into shaping me. I realized that state by state, our country was beginning to gnaw away at the hemline of cannabis prohibition. However, the states where freedoms were being doled out, plant based healthcare was being prioritized, and generational wealth was being created did not have demographics that looked like those of the states who chose to focus on filling prison beds with heads instead.

As an immigration attorney, I witnessed first-hand the disparities between communities where individuals were able to partake in the benefits of full adult use and medicinal cannabis markets in stark contrast to their counterparts in states with higher immigrant populations where cannabis laws moved slower and restitution often fell away from the conversation about legalization. What became painfully clear to me was that prohibition was marked by the propaganda, scandal, and cruelty of an unspoken marriage between private corporations and political agendas keen on doubling down on the misinformation surrounding cannabis, its value, and the perceived face of who used it. This left me with an urgent need to address the social injustices that had suddenly become quite obvious to me. It was then that I began to look closer at the intersectionality between race, prison and cannabis. I continued to see a recurring oddity, asking myself, "Why so many immigration detainees were brought into the system on cannabis-related charges, most of which resulted from minor, non-violent and non-trafficking arrests?"

The second fateful situation that brought me to cannabis came not only as a surprise, but as a swift blow, all too close to home, the type of unanticipated challenge that either makes or breaks the human spirit. Without warning, I was asked to help navigate the course of a close relative confronted with some cruel choices after learning of his child's diagnosis of epilepsy. He was being asked to choose between FDA approved drugs with potentially life threatening side effects or risking his freedom and family to seek out naturopathic remedies, including cannabis, in a state where cannabis was not legal. Advising someone I loved through the overwhelming landscape of inconsistent and unfair laws regarding who gets access to what medical care provided the push I needed to accelerate my curiosity about disparities, turning it into a ravenous passion for justice in the fight towards a national end to cannabis prohibition.

What I started to understand was that the inclusion of cannabis into conversations about saving our youth from the ills of drugs was an intentional conflation of concepts that had very little to do with one another and that none of it was driven by the medical community or even a sincere attempt to address the health and well being of Americans. On the contrary, the misinformation disseminated to the masses was a tiny part of a much more damaging plot to stifle undesirable communities while elevating and funding the wealth of a small group of power players who would benefit from the casualties of our nation's drug war.

The history of cannabis prohibition and the War on Drugs are so intricately tied to issues of wealth distribution, systematic racism, and politics that it is difficult to identify any valid origin that supports a legitimate reason that cannabis should ever have been banned. Wide spread national attitudes about cannabis legalization began to change as the eldest of my children was entering high school, a particularly daunting time for many parents. Change as we all know can be terrifying and I was not yet fully ready for it, did not quite know where my own convictions stood and certainly had not figured out how to reconcile the changes both in society and within myself that would result in a radical modification of how I parented around the subjects of pharmaceutical versus unapproved drugs.

Ironically, it was a similar fear of the unknown, one that attached itself to the insecurities of parenting, that had helped ramp up prohibition to begin with. By historical accounts, a shift in who was beginning to use cannabis recreationally facilitated an easy platform from which to bolster the narrative that cannabis was a "dangerous drug." During the early 1970's, some factions were concerned with the rise of young, white, college students experimenting with the plant and felt something drastic should be done to turn that tide. It should come as no surprise then that five decades later, popular American sentiment about how cannabis and drugs,in general, should be treated would be intertwined with a desire to extend compassion for those suffering from the "opioid crisis," a compassion that seemed to be strangely absent during the earlier "crack epidemic."

The third fateful situation that thrust me into the path of cannabis advocacy came with my own frustration and disillusionment. Unsatisfied with the ever growing list of inequities plaguing legalization, I sought out fellow attorneys, specifically Black attorneys, with which to begin the very real and critical conversations that needed to take place about the lack of diversity within the industry. To my shock, there were very few Black attorneys having those conversations on a national level, and even fewer were present in the places where key decisions about the framework of the industry were being made. Disgusted by the lack of presence and concerned by the possibility that the industry would be built without any true redress of the systematic devastation caused by the failed War on Drugs, I set out to build a network and resource for those seeking equity, inclusion and reparative justice in cannabis.

Headed by a diverse pool of Black voices within the legalization space and the allies that recognized the need for this movement, the National Association of Black Cannabis

Lawyers (NABCL), was born. Together we formed an alliance of attorneys and advocates from around the country with a mission of ensuring that the federal cannabis landscape does not continue to fail those most adversely affected by a prohibition that should never have been.

The task of building the NABCL has been an amazing exercise in self reflection and learning to be comfortable being uncomfortable. I often feel far out of my depth, but I am surrounded by an incredible team of people who value the impact of our efforts. The most important members of my team are the five humans whom I have been charged with guiding into their own life journey. From the outside looking in, I imagine it seemed as if overnight I went from "just say no" to "legalize all fifty." But in reality, the changes in my personal beliefs were actually the result of an openness to a reeducation concerning the science and history of cannabis, an understanding that the lines between heroes and villains are not always obvious and a willingness to listen to the whys of others. Because it is there within the stories that we sometimes learn our own truths and in the process discover how we can change the ending.

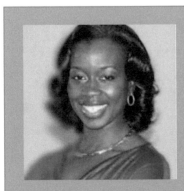

Natacha Andrews, Esq
www.nabcl.com
info@nabcl.com
Linkedin: Natacha Delinois Andrews
Learn more about Natacha at www.courageincannabis.com:

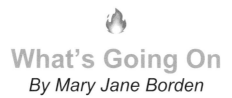

What's Going On
By Mary Jane Borden

What's going on? A simple query. These three words, though, from the iconic Marvin Gaye still resonate today—fifty years after the song and record album by that name topped the music charts in 1971. The escalating Vietnam War and the protest movement that vehemently opposed it inspired the lyrics. Exponential increases in US military casualties and incursions into other countries troubled Gaye, as did the killings of four students by the Ohio National Guard at Kent State University. In the song, he questions the need for violence, brutality, prejudice, and hate.

Marvin Gaye was a product of the 1960s: peace, love, understanding…and marijuana. The laid-back atmosphere in the Motown Record's recording studio was legendary and often brought on by the constant smoke that encircled Gaye and other musicians. To the surprise of no one, "What's Going On" was a creative product of cannabis. Barry Gordy, the owner of that record label, outright rejected the song, calling it the worst thing he had ever heard in his life. He refused to release it. Undeterred, Gaye, one of Motown's most popular acts, responded by essentially going on strike. Gordy acquiesced, and the song was released.

The triumphant power of the lyrics of "What's Going On" lies in the larger lessons it teaches. Ambitious politicians often utilize war-like rhetoric to advance their causes. Wars have been declared to end poverty, cure cancer and fight drugs. They have been waged from Afghanistan to Iraq to Ukraine. Fifty years later, *not one worked.* Clearly, war is not the answer.

What does work? Gaye offers some clues. For one, love. Gaye may have been channeling the inspirational words of Dr. Martin Luther King, Jr., who said something along the lines of hate cannot drive out hate; only love can do that. Gaye also decries discrimination based on physical appearance and police brutality at political protests. Instead, he repeatedly spread words like "talk to me" to "bring some understanding here today." Communication is key to diffusing conflict.

It takes courage to believe in your work, tackle controversial issues, and defy your boss. Marvin Gaye did all of that. That cannabis intertwines his story makes it all the more profound.

Today, the lyrics of the song "What's Going On" and its message remain relevant. The album is recognized as one of the most important musical works of the Twentieth Century. Bruce Springsteen called it a masterpiece. Because of this song, Marvin Gaye was inducted into the Rock and Roll Hall of Fame and received a Grammy Lifetime Achievement Award. A half-century later, the record still ranks number one on Rolling Stone's 500 Greatest Albums of All Time.

Overall, "What's Going On" illustrates what courage, conviction, and cannabis can do triumphantly.

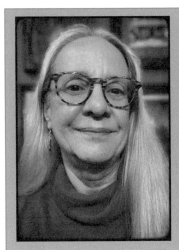

Mary Jane Borden
Author, Graphic artist, Journalist
CannabinArt.com
maryjaneborden@gmail.com
FB:@Mary Jane Borden

Learn more about Mary Jane
at www.courageincannabis.com:

From Stoner To Triumphant TribuNARY

By Michelle Nary

I was born on December 5, 1963, into a cannabis-friendly household during the biggest blizzard of the year. My father was as "OG" as they come. I've been a "stoner" since high school and for most of my life. I've been an activist and advocate from my home state of Ohio to Michigan, to Florida, and to anyone who would listen.

As a young teen, I discovered my parents smoked cannabis. I knew it was against the law and that if anyone found out, it would split our six-member family apart. "That '70s Show" was really my life—the difference being my parents were the ones smoking it, and in the living room, not in the basement. I didn't really have many friends in high school, but when I told a couple of people about the cannabis at my house, my friend count grew.

My dad had a lot of friends as well. I remember when they all jumped on their motorcycles and went to Ann Arbor, Michigan, to attend the first of many "Hash Bash" festivals. Since then, I have stood in solidarity on those same steps many times with other Michigan activists, advocates, educators and patients.

My mother quit smoking cannabis the day she found out that I had started.

My father taught me to clean cannabis using a can he called "The Great Divide." It was a large coffee can with a removable screen inside that separated seeds and stems. Dad then used it as a prototype for a renewable system made from pieces of screen, duct tape and a coffee can with the bottom cut out and the lid placed on the bottom for easy emptying. My Grammy taught me how to make canna tea from the stems of cannabis.

I used to tell my friends that I was going to go to Amsterdam and be a judge at the cup. I went to Amsterdam in 2005 with my dad. Since then, I have visited nearly every "coffee" shop, and I have been to several "High Times Cannabis Cup" events, but I have never been asked to be a judge; I think there's still time!

Out of four children, all have blue eyes, but only one chose cannabis. I wish I knew how many joints I've rolled in my lifetime; rolling dad's ten a day for thirty years, plus five a day for myself. I utilized cannabis illegally for many years to help me relax and sleep. I sometimes worked two jobs, one to pay bills and the second to afford cannabis.

I got a job working for a couple of lawyers and ended up being accused of a check-cashing crime that I didn't commit. It took me two and a half years under court supervision to prove my innocence. During that time, I was unable to use cannabis. I was told, "The court cannot have you using drugs under supervision. We can get you all the help you need."

The threat of jail time was all the "help" I needed. I quit on the spot without incident, and three months later, I expected to test negative for THC, but I was wrong. That's when I found out that my body makes endocannabinoids and that I would never test completely negative. I did not smoke for two and a half years. While I was under supervision, I was able to get my CDL training and license. I was able to go over the road driving a semi and to come back periodically for court. After I was found not guilty, I told my court supervisor, "The only thing I was guilty of was using cannabis and speeding."

One sunny afternoon in September of 2003, I was rear-ended at a high rate of speed by a semi/trailer while I was operating a fully loaded semi/trailer. I received no obvious injuries, but my body refused to heal. Turns out that I have an issue with letters and numbers. I am HLA-B27 positive, meaning I have the human leukocyte antigen B27 protein attached to my white blood cells, which gives me a greater risk of developing certain autoimmune disorders, arthritis and spondyloarthritis, to name a few. This all impeded my progress.

In 2009, I spent my days volunteering as a contributing editor to a Facebook page called "Grannies for Grass." I would scan the web for anything relevant, anything new regarding cannabis and the ways people were using it to find relief. I met a living angel named Robin Fisher. I didn't know it then, but she would be my "canna sensei" in that she taught me almost everything I know about how to add cannabis to just about anything.

Robin taught me the value of the CBD flower. I had no experience with it before. It made my body feel so much more without pain. I still got relief but without the heavy buzz.

Concerning THC, I told Robin there was no amount of cannabis that could make me feel like I was drunk, as I had heard some people have that feeling if they utilize too much, too fast. I can tell you from personal experience that, for me, a gram and a half is too much. Thank goodness for black pepper oil! Swishing black pepper with warm water around my mouth helped to lessen the heavy feeling and bring me back to clarity.

We were always educating, even traveling cross country to educate voters at Florida Hempfest near Tampa. In 2015, I was invited to an event in Michigan where I was chosen to be the director of all US chapters of "Grannies for Grass." We had a chapter in every state and a group page for every chapter as well, so I reviewed and shared information on over one hundred pages. Robin was the deputy director.

There was a time in my life when I was stuck flat in my bed for four months, unable to walk well or climb stairs without excruciating pain. I had a live-in caregiver whose responsibilities included caring for my father and our home. Suddenly, he was stuck caring for me full-time as well. My spine had collapsed on my nerves. I tried everything to relieve my pain. I'm grateful for pain medication allergies because I know that otherwise, as bad as I hurt, I would've been another statistic addicted to painkillers. I was so depressed that suicide was never far from my mind, and if it wasn't for the need to care for my dog, MerceNary, I would've given up.

I finally jumped through enough hoops with the internationally renowned Cleveland Clinic hospital to potentially get an appointment with the neurological surgeon. We had a conversation on the phone, and I asked, "So why can't I have surgery?"

He said, "We don't do elective surgery on drug addicts." When I asked who's a drug addict, he said, "You use marijuana."

I said, "Yes, I do. I'm not allergic to it, and it works. It's also 2017. Cannabis is legal in our state. Is this your opinion or the opinion of the Cleveland Clinic?" He told me it was the opinion of the clinic, and I asked, "That so? Kindly refer to my medical record dated six weeks ago when the clinic did surgery on me. It was a life-and-death cyst removal from my jawline. You don't know what you're talking about. I'll speak to your boss, please. You're fired."

My triple spinal fusion was done at the main campus of the hospital on March 8, 2017. My in-hospital stays have been very short, with few pharmaceutical interventions. In 2021 on April 20, I had cervical surgery to replace a vertebra. I had another lumbar surgery on July 16 of the same year. I also had a complete lumbar fusion on May 6, 2022. That was a forty-eight-hour stay. Thirty-six hours, in I was utilizing only Tylenol. No additional pain medication. I climbed the stairs easily with the therapist, and I walked laps most of the night before I was discharged.

A little dab will do me.

CBD is an incredible helper to THC! Between the two, I can give most pain a good kick out of my body, easing my anxiety about the pain, and that leads to having the ability to *move*. This is critical for me as a diabetic that also has multiple inflammatory disorders. Being free of pain and free of the fear of pain is life-changing and enables me to walk. And walking helps me to get better, without the side effects of pharmaceuticals. I can dance again!

On November 6, 2018, in Roscommon, Michigan, I voted to allow recreational cannabis in the state of Michigan. I had moved there early that year as a medical refugee to continue to be able to stay pharmaceutical-free and also to do so naturally. As it happened, I lived in a city that I had been visiting with my friend for many years. Houghton

Lake, Michigan, appeared in my past many times before I met my sponsors, my caregivers, and my family.

I was at a music festival in Southwestern Ohio, and I heard a band on stage. They were singing a song about cannabis. My dog, MerceNary, and I went to see what it was all about. As I watched from the field, some distance away, one of the band members started telling me how cannabis helped him heal, how he had multiple sclerosis, and cannabis oil helped him with his activities of daily living by relieving the pain. I was stunned. I yelled, "Me too!" and we went closer.

By the end of his speech, I was standing on the rail next to an older man I did not know. When the band set was over, I was told to come find them to talk. I had a conversation with the gentleman on the rail before I left, and it turned out that he knew my caregivers, Kristina Bailey, Jennifer Cook, and Nikki Abbey. I'm not sure which one of us was more surprised, and he blurted out, "I have been your guardian angel!" It turned out that he knew where all the flowers originated, which helped to keep me sane and pain-free.

From the time my father came out of the service in 1962 until he turned seventy-five in 2017, he was a cannabis user. At the age of seventy-five, he was put in a nursing home, and the cannabis use stopped. My father became unbearable with the nursing staff.

At one point, I was secretly dosing him with THC so he would continue to get the medicine he needed to make him tolerable. Once the nurses found out, they made me stop due to being a federally funded establishment. My father was a veteran, and when I shared the circumstances with his veteran buddies, they made a plan because veterans stick together. There was a line of veterans waiting to visit my father to take turns giving him what he needed, so I wouldn't be in trouble. Unfortunately, he became unable to swallow and never received that help. My father passed away at the age of seventy-seven, and for the first time in fifty-seven years, he was sober.

I found my cannabis courage in educating medical staff non-stop and by demanding quality care in spite of being considered a "drug addict." I used cannabis to quit drinking alcohol, stop smoking cigarettes, stop taking a ton of pharmaceuticals and so I could get to a place where I could actually meditate. I can only speak from my experience and pray others find their path.

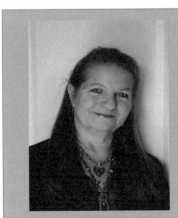

Michelle Nary
michellenary@gmail.com
Mothers Cannabis:
www.facebook.com/mothercann
TribuNary Holistic Consultations:
www.facebook.com/THConsultations

Learn more about Michelle
at www.courageincannabis.com:

The True Spark of DOPEness

By LaKesha Randle

Hi there. I am LaKesha Randle, and I am a Sickle Cell Warrior!

Sickle cell anemia is an inherited disorder that affects the shape of red blood cells, which carry oxygen to all parts of the body. When my body is stressed in any way, my red blood cells that shaped like crescent moons, which can slow or block blood flow in the body causing extreme pain. There's no cure for most people with sickle cell anemia (stem cell and bone marrow transplants are now options but not a guaranteed cure). Treatments mainly focus on pain relief and specifically opioid medications.

Sickle cell for me at least, has been a lifelong battle that I now know is fought best spiritually and mentally. What do I mean by that? From the time I had my first memorable pain crisis and being brought up in church believing in Jesus Christ, I was taught God never gives us more than we can bear. I believed that with everything in me in my youth, and it gave me a fearless personality because my way of thinking was that if God allowed me to have sickle cell it's because he knew I could endure a large amount of pain and survive. I felt special, like I must be some kind of super human! I fight spiritually by praying and worshiping through the pain, reading, memorizing certain bible scriptures, and I use to post them around my hospital room. I fight mentally now by keeping busy doing activities that help distract me from my pain, but will help create a better future for myself and my daughter. I sometimes journal about my pain and do artwork to help express myself which helps combat things on the mental/emotional side.

I will tell you from my experience in my thirty-two years of life that I have had thousands of pain crises, twenty-nine surgeries, countless seizures, and many other complications. I had strokes at a ridiculously young age and ended up on a walker, all before starting my freshman year in high school. Before I knew it, due to the bleeding in my brain and muscle weakness, I found myself on my deathbed at least three times, caught up in a cycle of daily pain and consuming high doses of pain medication to combat it. This ultimately led to something called opioid dependency.

For patients suffering painful, life-threatening illnesses, such as sickle cell, opioid dependency is commonly known to exist. I was informed about this by multiple doctors when I lived in Ohio and even now here in Florida. They normalized this addiction and the destruction it played in my life. After all, it was coming from a doctor, so it must be okay. Spiritually and Mentally it wasn't, I was losing my Faith and will to survive, becoming addicted to the feeling of being numb and escaping pain and reality through prescription. I remember being angry with God for what I once considered a superhuman strength became just pain and suffering. I started to pray less and depend more on my medication and the doctors although I still believed in God, I no longer felt special. At this time I was taking ridiculous amounts of Oxycontin, Oxycodone™, Dilaudid™ and morphine at higher and higher doses every year. After years of living life highly medicated constantly, my personality started to change. I was no longer me; I was a shell of myself walking around and barely existing. No longer living or feeling, I was numb, a walking zombie!

This period in my life is where I believe my faith in God was tested tremendously. The devil thought he had me completely won over, But God didn't allow it to take me out. Despite that, however, I felt alone.

My relationships with my family suffered quite a bit. I have a brother, Broderick, with the same genetic illness, and at times I would not even reach out to him. In my heavily sedated, medicated, altered mind, I believed he was not going through the same health complications and could not possibly understand my problems.Although we had some similar experiences with sickle cell while growing up, we had some completely different experiences with the disease as we became older.

I fell deep into depression and isolated myself from those closest to me, including my mother and brothers, who only wanted to help me. My relationship with my mom, Claudette, was negatively affected. She tried to help by being present, loving, caring, patient, supportive, prayerful, and always in my corner no matter what happened. Although I could not always clearly communicate to her or my brothers what my internal dilemmas were. Why? It was a combination of all the issues of addiction and dependency, something I did not understand myself.

Shockingly, I became a mother while in this unclear state of mind. I was twenty-three, and this is when the support and the love of my family kicked into overdrive. My brother Broderick introduced cannabis to me as a healthier option hoping it could help me see that I was not alone, that, now, there were sickle cell pain management options available other than just opioids.

I was resistant for a long time. Whether it was the addiction to the pills, the disbelief in the plant or a combination of the two, it took several years for me to decide to remove myself from the grasp of opioids and actually give cannabis a chance.

I had to grow and learn from the problems that affected me mentally. I have never been in a domestically abusive relationship with a person. However, in theory, that is what my relationship with sickle cell and opioid dependency felt like. A codependent abusive relationship that I literally saw no way to get out of.

As soon as I thought I was doing better and becoming independent, the opioids would pull me back over and over again. I believed I could not find pain relief without them, that no other medication could take care of me the way opioids could. They had a hold on me, and it took faith and pure determination to break free. I'm happy to report my faith in God has been restored and back to feeling superhuman again! I truly believe that my life serves a purpose and if that purpose is to simply tell my truth, then that's what i'll do. My truth gives God all the glory because the doctors, medical field, some teachers, some family members, even myself counted me out years ago but God counted me in. I'm so grateful and humbled, you never gave up on me!#TimeWell$pent

Today, I can honestly say cannabis has helped me in multiple ways to treat my sickle cell and opioid dependency. With my use of cannabis in many forms, I'm now on the lowest dose of opioids I've ever been on in my life. This plant continues to help me daily, and I thank God I do not look like everything I have been through because sickle cell has put me through hell and back!

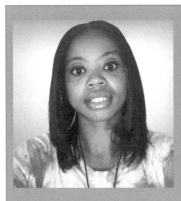

LaKesha Randle
lakesharandle27@gmail.com
IG:lakesha_scw
FB: LaKesha Faith'sMom Randle

Learn more about LaKesha
at www.courageincannabis.com:

The Time Is Now
By Frederika Easley

We come into the world advocating selfishly for our needs. We are then beaten into submission by societal norms. It is my hope that, as we age, we can get back to prioritizing our "feel good."

If you need to balance out, cannabis can help.

If you need to heal, cannabis can help.

If you need to release and unwind, cannabis can help.

If you are looking to quiet your mind, cannabis can help.

If your appetite needs awakening, yes, cannabis can help.

The stories in this book show the many benefits of cannabis and showcase the need for more research and normalization.

The time for Black, Latinx and Indigenous people and communities to claim what is owed and to use cannabis to repair our collective harm is now. We must take it!

Taking from a statement by the prolific American writer James Baldwin, he shared that there is never a time in the future in which we will work out our salvation, in contrast, the challenge is in the moment, THE TIME IS ALWAYS NOW!

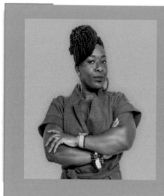

Frederika McClary Easley
Director of Strategic Initiatives at The People's Ecosystem
Host of The People Are Blunt Podcast
http://thepeoplesecostystem.com/about-us
IG: @Klassik84
Linkedin: Frederika McClary Easley
Learn more about Frederika at www.courageincannabis.com

Escaping the Invisible Box
By Tonica Spicer Combs

***Content Advisory: This chapter will discuss experiences of domestic and emotional abuse. Please engage in self-care as you read this chapter.

When you look at me, what do you see? Honestly, I would like to think most people who know me see a genuinely kind, funny and caring person. But there was one person in my life that reduced me down to just a mere superficial aesthetic. He only liked how my hair and skin looked, the way my body was built. At least that's what he told me when he began stuffing me into that shallow man-made box.

I fucking hated that box.

It's the place he would always shove me into when I became more than he wanted. When I decided to be myself, speak up about things that bothered me or speak on things that I liked or disliked or anything else for that matter.

That same cramped-ass box he would smush and contort me into when he never respected me enough to be completely honest with me.

It was that dusty, broken-down teeny, tiny-ass box I knew I didn't belong in. I never belonged in. But someone that I thought loved me put me there in that box with all of their emotional and mental abuse.

Lies, manipulation, theft and betrayal are all forms of abuse. Please do not let anyone tell you otherwise. It is the most insidious kind of abuse. The kind that slowly crept its way into my own thoughts over time and was so warped and twisted that it made me look at myself completely differently.

The isolation, the gaslighting, walking on eggshells just to keep the peace was insane. I truly felt like I was losing my mind. He treated me more like a child needing to ask permission rather than his spouse. The outrageous accusations and arguments leading in circles, never finding a resolution, were mentally and emotionally exhausting. I was so drained, depressed and in my own head that I couldn't see my children were each going through their own unique struggles.

The abuse I endured over many years took me away from being a good mom, which was the only thing I ever wanted to be in life. The anxiety of worrying about him being angry at something I did or didn't do... Just hearing his car pull up when he came home from work made me sick to my stomach.

I was discouraged from working, having my own car, or even having access to finances because I was told I was irresponsible. I was questioned about the most innocent things, berated when I didn't measure up with thinly veiled "jokes," and continually disrespected and betrayed over and over again for years.

I was isolated from family and friends and discouraged from making new friends. The one person I trusted to love, honor and cherish me was the one person who devastated me to my core. The constant fear of losing who I was and not being able to think for myself was a very scary place to be.

I retreated into myself and began "self-medicating" by overeating and consuming alcohol almost daily. My weight ballooned up over three hundred pounds, and the heavier I became physically, the heavier my mind felt too.

Once the suicidal thoughts began, I knew I had to seek professional help. I was so glad when I finally found a therapist because I honestly felt like I was losing my mind. She told me that we could never "fix" things because he was never honest or forthcoming with the horrible things he'd done.

He used to blame me for everything wrong in his life when the cause of the chaos in our lives was him. My therapist told me, "He's a broken man, and you can't fix him."

I reached out to everyone close to me for help, but they didn't know what to do. I reached out to our church, which was absolutely no help at all, unfortunately. I even began reaching out to strangers on social media, desperate for help, but without evidence of physical abuse, no one would get involved or knew how to help. I felt hopeless.
But then, thankfully, the turning point in my life and my salvation to breaking my way out of that cramped-ass little box came with beginning the use of medical cannabis.

In 2019, I thought I would give cannabis a try to help alleviate my symptoms of PTSD. I got my card as soon as the program was available. And it has helped turn my life around tremendously!

At the time of receiving my card, I was on three different prescription pharmaceuticals for depression, anxiety and PTSD due to the traumatic, toxic marriage mentioned above. Those medications never seemed to help. Instead, they just made me feel like a zombie and like I couldn't grasp everyday life.

Amazingly, after filling my first prescription of medical cannabis, I quit all pharmaceuticals. And though it worked for me, I am, in no way, encouraging anyone to stop taking their medication, especially if it works for you. Always consult your physician. But for me, the clarity cannabis gave me has been absolutely eye-opening.

For me, consuming cannabis completely began to open my mind and relax me in ways I hadn't experienced in years. It brought me so much clarity and self-reflection. It helped release the anxiety I felt and slowed down those nasty, intrusive thoughts and feelings brought on by being shoved down into that box for so many years.

The more I medicated with cannabis, the more I'd begun to feel like I could think for myself again and that I was strong enough to go out in the world and function and provide a good life for myself and my children.

With every toke of cannabis and each edible I consumed, I laughed harder and cried a lot less. My mood lifted, and I felt more balanced than I ever had in my life. I stopped letting that negativity and hurt break me down. I listened to my family and friends when they told me how strong they all knew I was, and I started to actually believe it and started to feel like myself again.

I found a great job, got my own car and finally gained access to an attorney to file for divorce, and I can't even begin to describe how incredibly freeing it felt!

I used to be so embarrassed and afraid to talk about what my ex-husband did to me and how much it affected me. But during this journey of healing, I realized that it doesn't matter how he feels about me discussing my experience. If he wanted people to think he was a good person, then he should have been a good person.

Cannabis helped and is continuing to help heal my mind, body and spirit. It has gotten such a bad reputation since the 1937 racist propaganda, but I see positive change on the horizon for this truly magnificent plant and hope it continues to help and heal many others in the world.
I am living proof that it can be life-changing, and I will definitely continue to sing its praises for many years to come!

***If you or someone you know is experiencing domestic abuse, help is available:
Text the National Domestic Violence Hotline by texting "START" to 88788 or call 1-800-799-SAFE (7233) or chat online at https://www.thehotline.org/
Text the Crisis Text Line by texting HOME to 741741. (www.crisistextline.org**)**

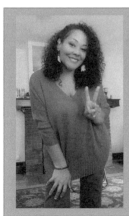

Tonica Spicer Combs

tonicacombs@gmail.com

Learn more about Tonica
at www.courageincannabis.com

Defining Courage
By Jamie Lynn Dodd

Denial, anger, bargaining, depression, and acceptance. We've all heard of the stages of grief endured in the act of losing someone or something meaningful or significant, and chances are, most of you reading this have suffered through this process more than once in this lifetime already. I never anticipated being diagnosed with a life threatening disease, to be a grieving process as well.

My life was what could be considered normal for a 14-year-old girl until the morning of March 14, 2005. I was vivacious, full of life and ignorantly naive to any real problems this life could inflict on a person, as most teenagers blissfully are. My mom noticed my joyful bouncing energy was turning to irritability, insatiable thirst and hunger and then crashing into fatigue. That brisk March morning, my mom scheduled a doctor's appointment for a check up. My world as I knew it came to a screeching halt, was promptly flipped on its head, and irrevocably changed forever.

I was diagnosed as a brittle Type-1 diabetic in one single moment in my doctor's office when my blood glucose levels read nine times higher than that of a normal glucose reading. Hospitalized for the week that followed, I learned that a blood sugar of 900 induced a coma for most diabetics, if not death. I will never know how or why I was functioning with complete normality when my health was "critical" by definition, but to this day I believe it to be the epitome of my mentality in dealing with this vicious and unforgiving disease.

"Denial: The action of declaring something to be untrue". My denial began the second I was admitted to the hospital directly from the doctor's office, whether I realized it or not. In my teenage brain (and sometimes my adult one, too) there was no possible way I could be as fragile, weak or sick as the doctors asserted I was. No matter what I was told or learned in my diagnosis, I truly believed my health and life wouldn't be affected much by any of this and that I could continue just the same as I had before that fateful morning. While most teenagers have the innocent luxury of simply trying to figure out who they are in the world as they're discovering it to be, most of my teenage years were spent in the bed of the ICU discovering how fragile life can truly be, yet still never fully accepting that this was my lot in life. I became reckless in those first few years and my health suffered.

Anger, bargaining, depression... These stages of the grieving process all seemed to melt and morph together as a super-monster of self-loathing and bitterness towards my disease. My body had ultimately failed me in this life, that is how I've felt over the last two decades. Is this illness something a person can ever truly "accept"? Are anger and depression not normal, if not rational, feelings to have when enduring a disease that is relentlessly painful and exhausting? How would any person of any walk of life handle a diagnosis of suffering that would last until their last breath? To sit with these thoughts and questions daily consumed and reduced me, eventually. Gone was the girl I described as vivacious and full-of-life. She had been replaced with a bitter version of herself that hated what had become of her: a victim of chronic illness.

The most pivotal moment of my journey with Diabetes was learning about medical cannabis. Managing the physical aspect of my disease is an act that comes as second nature now. The frequently drastic swings of my blood sugars, the endless sticks from needles of all shapes and sizes, constantly being "sick" because of my depleted immune system, and the daily exhaustion and pain are just a few of the physical issues I've endured.

When I first had exposure to regulated, quality medical marijuana, I found the relief I was searching for in this plant. I was desperate for a better quality of life. I knew this plant would never cure me, or rid my body of the problems I had, but I hoped that it would alleviate the physical struggles I faced daily. And it has, for the most part.

For years, I have struggled with managing the mental and emotional roller coaster of this disease, because of the lack of choice that I have. Everything about this disease is a matter of life or death and that can be a hard pill to swallow. While I had always hoped that cannabis would provide relief to my physical symptoms I never once realized or expected the profound impact it would have on my mental health as well.

In most aspects of life as adults we hear that mentality is "half the battle", this statement is applicable to so many instances we endure in this world. But when the mentality of daily life is knowing that you must endure or cease to live, that's a recipe for some wild emotions and feelings that no one can outrun or hide from; these feelings always catch you eventually. So, while I think that the best I can ever do is to keep those feelings of anger and depression at a minimal and manageable level, I know that I can find solace from those emotions through cannabis.

What this beautiful plant medicine has done is re-instill a certain kind of hope that I was so desperate to feel for so long. While many would argue that the "physical" benefits I experience from cannabis greatly outweigh the "mental" benefits, I would beg to differ. There has been great victory from the relief of physical woes this disease has brought forth. After years of cannabis use, my neuropathy that could be relentless at times has almost completely subsided and my weakened immune system will hold its own from time to time. These are not small feats.

But I can't, and won't, ever be able to continue my battle without maintaining the way I think and feel about it all, as well. If it weren't for cannabis, the "dark" days I sometimes have would last so much longer than they do. Those feelings can be terrifying when they consume and take over, and I can't think about what I would do if I didn't have this plant to calm my thoughts, to soothe the worries and anxieties I feel. Even medicating before appointments with my therapist (which I find crucial to living with diabetes) allows me to feel more relaxed and comfortable in sharing thoughts that can otherwise be difficult to say out loud.

This plant, with all its taboos and stigmas, has given me back a part of my life that I had lost hope for ever having again. I'm not sure I will ever fully experience a feeling of complete "acceptance" when it comes to this disease, knowing all it has taken from me thus far. But any acceptance I do have has been birthed and reared entirely by medical marijuana. The hope it has instilled is the fuel my mind, body and soul feed off to keep fighting this fight, for my children and partner, for my parents and siblings, for all those people who have stood by my side and fought with me in this battle over the years.

The people who refuse to believe in the power of this plant haven't felt the exasperation and desperation of a person living with a chronic illness, and more than likely never will until it is them or a loved one around them fighting a battle of their own.

And while my own story has moments that have caused denial, sadness, and anger within me, the entirety of this journey I've been on with Type-1 Diabetes is nothing short of awe-inspiring. This body of mine has been one of the most phenomenal displays of physical and emotional strength that I ever have and ever will see in my lifetime. The most humbling concept to accept is that strength does not always have to come from within when dealing with the battle diabetes inflicts. And even though I get lost or stray from my strength sometimes, I've come to realize that it's okay to draw my strength from this plant when I cannot muster it myself.

Courage, by definition, is the ability to do something that frightens one. It is strength in the face of pain or grief. Every morning that I wake up and brace myself for that day's battle against diabetes is nothing short of a courageous act. And because of cannabis, that battle seems less daunting than it was two decades ago, and I find myself regaining ground back to that girl who could be described as "vivacious" and "full of life", daily. My courage in this fight now exudes grace and elegance, and my hope remains rigid and intact all because of this plant. And because of these qualities instilled in my core, I know that no matter what, cannabis has forever changed the way I wage my war against this treacherous disease. Because of this plant, I finally see this battle for what it truly is: beautiful.

This is dedicated to ones that have stood diligently by my side in my fight with this disease. Most importantly, this is for my parents: my mom and dad, Tim and Cathy, who have been molding and shaping me for 32 years into the woman I am proud to be today, and the parents I've gained as bonuses, my stepmother and -father, Wendy and Jerry. If any of them has ever been scared at any point in the last two decades, they've never shown it. Their own displays of courage and grace in my diagnosis and disease have been a beacon of strength that have always shown me how to persevere. Especially my mother, who has always been the real-life M'Lynn Eatenon to my Shelby since the moment I was diagnosed. Mom, you are nothing short of a phenomenal woman, a force to be reckoned with, and hands down the most tenacious and terrifying woman I know. Thank you for showing me the true definition of a Bad-Ass and thank you for always being MY Steel Magnolia.

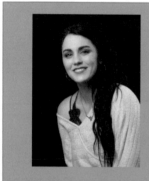

Jamie Lynn Dodd
jlynndodd@icloud.com
Linkedin: Jamie Lynn Dodd

Learn more about Jamie
at www.courageincannabis.com:

By Jane West

his is the decade of cannabis. By the end of the twenties, the vast majority of Americans will have access to a multitude of regulated cannabis products. Currently, both regulated and unregulated cannabis markets are booming, and countries are legalizing its use across the globe.

But who will be licensed to grow and sell the world billions of dollars of cannabis? Currently, the owners are generationally wealthy, white men operating Canadian publicly traded companies on American soil. It is completely unacceptable, especially considering how cannabis prohibition decimated generations of diverse communities with the war on drugs.

Action must be taken now. A new generation of cannabis activists demanding home grow rights and local business access to cultivation, processing and retail must start fighting today in order to end this decade with a semblance of equity.

Cannabis is for everyone, and the faces of entrepreneurial success in the sector should reflect that diversity. I'm talking about women-owned businesses, Black-owned businesses, and locally-owned businesses. We all need to fight for our right to own a piece of the future.

Cannabis is a plant that all should have the right to grow, purchase and consume as we see fit.

JANE WEST

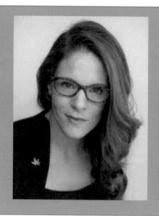

Jane West
CEO of Jane West Homegoods
Founder of Women Grow
www.janewest.com
jane@janewest.com

Learn more about Jane
at www.courageincannabis.com

Deeper Roots
By Rick Anstiss

The cannabis plant has been a part of my life since I was a teenager, becoming the only constant thing in my younger experimental years.

I found myself testing the waters of addiction. Whether it be alcohol or illicit drugs, cannabis was the one thing that spoke to my soul and helped me with my problems. The other things only compounded them.

As the medical program in Michigan began, the medicinal values that cannabis has always given me became more apparent. After losing my father to cancer in 2015, I realized my true calling in life. It was to explore this plant and learn as much about it as possible, then take that knowledge and help others.

In 2016, my wife told me to stop my roofing career and move forward with what my heart was telling me. So I did just that and became a caregiver in the Michigan Medical Marijuana Program. A Michigan caregiver is registered to grow twelve plants per patient for no more than five patients. The early stages of growing were hard and unforgiving. I found myself frustrated in learning how to properly navigate the growth of this plant. Still, I was eager to produce the best medicine possible within its genetics. As my knowledge grew, so did my awareness of the cannabinoids, particularly THC and CBD. They are all very important and very diverse in creating the entourage effect, the medicinal synergy of all the active components of the plant coming together.

I began to focus on the nutrients of growing the plant and the specific genetics of the strain I was working with.

Tediously, I wrote down feed charts and adjusted them according to my results. This takes time and lots of effort. Many cycles must be gone through before you can properly gather accurate data.

Through this process, I was also able to accentuate the terpenes—the medicinal essential oils—within this plant and adjust them according to the needs of my patients. Terpenes quite possibly could be the most important part of the entourage effect. I maintained this study for six years and helped many people, including myself, as I became confident in my pursuit of healing and its results. I now have great knowledge and experience in helping many debilitating diseases and ailments with flower, oil vapes, and edibles that I have created.

The Michigan Medical Marijuana Program allows a caregiver to grow, produce and create. So, we're not just farmers or agricultural scientists; we are the prescribing healer of what could be future pharmaceutical medicines companies might create. This responsibility weighs heavily on a caregiver of five patients.

It was an astronomical amount of work but much needed. I've had the ability to produce liter after liter of RSO (Rick Simpson Oil), a concentrated therapeutic form of cannabis. That has helped with the remission of many cancers, along with the relief of symptoms for things like Crohn's disease, multiple sclerosis and many other ailments.

I soon found the need for better access to medicine for patients and more networking among caregivers and patients. So I began to work with numerous local municipalities to figure out how to do this and gain acceptance of the idea.

I found comradery in the nearby town of Eau Claire, Michigan. I then hosted the first hemp and harvest festival the area had ever seen. This was in a community of fruit farmers that have been here for over one hundred and fifty years. It was a great success with over sixty vendors, twenty-five hundred attendees and a great expression of an early emerging industry.

Planning events slowly became my thing. I then reached out to the local golf course, Indian Lake Hills Golf Course, to begin the first cannabis golf outing in Southwest Michigan. I call it Hazey Holes. It is now in its fourth year with two hundred and forty golfers, fifty-four teams, and thirty-six industry-sponsored holes.

The sponsors set up booths at their sponsored hole t-box and hand out cannabis and swag and represent their brands as well as companies. I have had involvement with celebrities such as Tommy Chong, Calvin Johnson, Darren McCarty, Jim Belushi and Rob Dear, along with a few House representatives from my local districts. I even held a campaign fundraiser for our state attorney general, whom I've continued to work with. We have many state issues to resolve with cannabis, and she has assured me that we will get that work done.

In 2021, I was able to see a dream of mine begin to come true through all my networking ventures and efforts. I finally found the funding to start up my own micro-grow. A micro-grow is a licensed opportunity under our 2018 recreational law here in Michigan. The cannabis micro-grow license is and was set up for caregivers to find a way into the recreational market.

When this came to be, the owner of Hartford Speedway approached me to see if I had any interest in doing something cannabis related at the track. After pushing through all the red tape in the state and municipalities, my partners and I were able to move forward and gain a license. We became the fourth micro business in the State of Michigan.

It took about a year, but in 2022 we now had a five-thousand-square-foot building with a grow, a processing lab, and retail space. Since we were located in an event center, I was also able to hold events. We named the place Transcend, as this license was meant for caregivers to transcend into a regulated market.

My sole purpose in obtaining this license was to provide caregiver quality that far supersedes ninety percent of the recreational market and at a price point people can afford. It was also my goal to grow the plants in the manner that caregivers do, with medicine first in mind. Basically, top-shelf caregiver products, at a street price. Unfortunately, there are always challenges.

I began to see the motives of my funding partners, who took my complete business motto and every S.O.P. that I and others created. They then turned around and haggled with me to only give me one percent of the company.

This company did not last six months online. I walked away before their complete demise. Their mismanagement led to them restaffing the grow, retail, and management team. They simply had no idea how to operate what my buddy and I created. These guys were a shining example of the politics that fail us as citizens.

When this law was created in 2018, it was written that no out-of-state interest could get a license for two years. The first license didn't come online until November of 2019, practically two years later. They should have kept them out for ten years.

My partners were from Wisconsin and clearly had an agenda, just like "Big Cannabis" always does. That agenda almost never has anything to do with the health or well-being of others. I'll never stand behind anything that doesn't hold this plant in the right light.

I am currently working on achieving a meeting with the Attorney General's Office and the Cannabis Regulatory Agency (CRA) Director of the State, with hopes of explaining more about the already launched investigation on this company by the CRA. I want to explain how important it is for caregivers to be able to continue their entrepreneurship in this cannabis space. Big corporations can do whatever they want, but snubbing out the grassroots movement will never happen simply because people like myself and thousands of others will stand against it.

A total of 2,354,640 citizens of the State of Michigan voted yes for recreational use. And I'll bet my last dollar that ninety percent of them would never want to see a corporate takeover striving for citizens minimized in opportunity.

I am also co-owner of Big Cloud Universe, a collective of caregiver and patient-based event coordinators. In 2022, we were able to hold five outdoor camping caregiver-style events, with attendance for each in the thousands. That was a two-day event in Benton Harbor, Michigan, with attendance again in the thousands.

We are operating these festivals and events under the 2016 amendment of our medical law. That allows caregivers and patience to gather and network in a compassion club style. Since this area of our law is what some may consider gray, our collective has chosen to obtain a state license that allows us to be within the complete confines of the law.

Slowly the community and industry found themselves needing more activism.

In 2021, I was introduced to Ryan Bringold, a long-time activist of the people here in Michigan. He then introduced me to Amie Carter and Latrisha Matson. Collectively we began a group called Michigan Weedsters. In the beginning, this group was not a lobbying group but merely a collective of concerned patients, caregivers and citizens of the state. However, we blossomed into an organization that fought five House bills that were damaging to our medical program. We held an education dinner for House representatives and senators, along with two separate rallies at the Capitol steps and an annual bridge walk created by Ryan Bringold.

We definitely made our voices heard and took a solid stand at the state level. This fight will continue until we have safe and easy access for all medical patients in the State of Michigan.

In 2023, there will be a much more proactive approach as the new class of representation for the state has arrived, many of whom added their support and interest in handling matters within the cannabis space. This is where we hold them accountable.

Michigan leaders will continue to defend the laws that we created through citizen-driven petitions and voting initiatives. The House and Senate need a three-fourths vote to overturn or amend the recreational law, Proposition One. We will provide the House and Senate the proper information to make the right decisions for the people. The previous House bills that have been presented were based on fear, lies and deception.

This year through my events and activism, I was able to meet the band Mendo Dope. They are a culture-vibe musical group that also grows cannabis recreationally in Mendocino County, California. I have had them at basically every event this year. We recently did a project together, and they wrote a track for me to use with my activism. I named it "Deeper Roots."

"This is who I am. I will never change. I'm gonna stand my ground, helping' those in pain. I do this for my people; that's why I speak the truth. They don't understand our culture; they're just corporate vultures. We got deeper roots." (Mendo Dope)

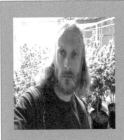

Rick Anstiss
anstiss421@gmail.com
https://www.facebook.com/rick.anstiss.10
IG: @mr._fungi420
Learn more about Rick
at www.courageincannabis.com:

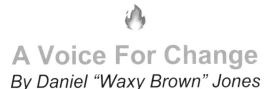

A Voice For Change
By Daniel "Waxy Brown" Jones

FREEZE! Put your hands up! You are under arrest!" I was surrounded by nine Drug Task Force Officers with nine guns pointed directly at my chest and back. Why? Because of prohibition.

After four years of festivals, cannabis and friends, the law caught up. Turns out cannabis and the distribution of the plant were still illegal in 2009. Daniel Jones, the fun-loving Deadhead Navy Veteran, was under arrest. And Waxy Brown was born.

When I was arrested for the distribution of a controlled substance (cannabis), I knew there was a major problem in this country, and having just served my country for eight years in the Navy, I knew it was time to serve my community again. Though, this time, my service came in the form of activism.

I spent two hundred and fifty-six days in jail, during which I continually refused a bond reduction in protest. I believed that a $300,000 bond for a plant was excessive, to say the least.

I began to try to change what was right in front of me. After serving five years on a very strict state probation, I ran for local government. I ran on a pro-legalization platform and trounced an eighteen-year incumbent three to one. Turns out cannabis is more popular than local politicians gave it credit for.

As I began to change local laws and conversations

surrounding cannabis, I found the opposition quite vocal. A local church raised a ruckus, and I was successfully ousted from office because of a bad law. In Missouri, the law states that if you have ever been convicted or plead guilty to a felony, you cannot hold public office. And I had, indeed, pled guilty in order to receive the probation deal.

My time in office was short (sixteen months) but effective and finished. We decriminalized an ounce or under of cannabis in Rolla, Missouri. I immersed myself in celebration for about ten minutes before I moved to the next project.

I wasn't finished. I couldn't just stop there. Cannabis became my path to activism. Activism became my passion. I had to act. I had to be heard. Our culture needed a voice that was loud and, in my humble opinion, *tie-dyed*.

I knew I had so much more to say. With the help of an OG Hippy who owned a classic rock radio station, Waxy Brown found a home and a microphone that reached the masses, and "Waxy Brown's Flower Power Hour" on KKID 92.9FM launched. Every Wednesday, we provide two hours of cannabis talk radio that is ten percent comedy and ninety percent cannabis education.

I couldn't do it without a team as waxy as I am. Tim Harms, Justin Trowbridge and Steve Wheeler hold down the ship with me. Having four different voices with four different perspectives is the magic behind the show.

From the green wave to the airwaves, we are advocating for our beautiful plant from a little old rock'n'roll station in the middle of America. It's what we do now. We stay *waxy* every Wednesday from 3pm to 5pm CST. It's still a fight, but it's in our ring now, our turf.

Stay waxy. Always.

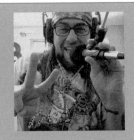

Daniel "Waxy Brown" Jones
www.waxybrownsflowerpowerhour.com
danieljonesforrolla@gmail.com

Learn more about Waxy
at www.courageincannabis.com:

My Strange And Wonderfully Weird Life

By Rebecca Stanforth

Being brought up by a single dad in the 80s and 90s was a strange time. My dad is still both a cannabis advocate and a martial arts instructor. I felt the odd combinations of stigma and respect for him while growing up. Back then, especially in his generation, he was called a hippie.

My dad did not hire childcare. He couldn't afford it. From a young age, I went everywhere with him. Electrical job sites during the day, martial arts studio in the evenings. Taking classes and learning martial arts was just my life. It wasn't a choice or an option.

We went on vacations but not normal family vacations. He took me to meditation retreats to meet and learn from people in different fields of mind/body alternative medicine. He took me to Buddhist and Hindu temples to learn, meditate, and pray. Dancing and chanting mantras in the Hindu temple is one of my favorite childhood memories. I had an amazing, wonderful childhood but a weird one. Is it any wonder I grew up to be just as strange and wonderfully weird as my father?

As the 90s was the time of "the war on drugs," the D.A.R.E. programs were heavy in my schools. In fifth grade, I was one of the winners in my school in a statewide essay writing contest. The theme was "Dare to Keep Kids Off Drugs." As an adult looking back, I wonder if it was my writing skills or my story.

I don't remember what exactly I wrote, but I wrote about what I knew. My mom was a recovering drug addict. She had lost custody of me when I was three, and that's why I was raised by my dad. I knew my mom struggled with mental health issues but didn't understand what that meant. Just that my mom was a "mentally ill recovering drug addict." I also knew a lot about drugs and their effects from both my parents and through attending Narcotics Anonymous meetings with my mom starting at five years old. I heard from addicts themselves long before I entered the D.A.R.E. program.

I also knew that my father didn't believe cannabis should be lumped in with other drugs. He said it had healing benefits and properties. He said it could be used to make healthy, environment-friendly products. He said it was medicine. Still, I understood, at age ten, that my father could be arrested and put in jail for having this medicine.

At the essay contest banquet, each winner got to read their essay at a podium while everyone had dinner. The police departments that promoted the D.A.R.E. program were present.

The beginning of my cannabis story started when that ten-year-old little girl walked up to that podium and read her story, terrified her father would be arrested for smelling like "his medicine." It was also the first time I spoke publicly about mental health. I saw my mom as a human trying to get better.

*****

Cannabis and Cancer

In early 2013, I left an abusive relationship. I had always known I had social anxiety, but it reached extreme levels. I was suffering from severe PTSD but didn't recognize it. I struggled to leave the house. My father's solution, as it had been for everything the previous thirteen years, was to return to martial arts classes and martial arts training. Slowly he wore me down. And I got better.

I wasn't just taking classes and teaching for my dad but also for the local school system. I was around instructors, elders, and people I love and have known since my earliest memories. People who helped raise the little girl who didn't have a normal mom and then lost her in 1999 to an MRSA infection. She was clean for the last ten years of her life.

Later in 2013, my father was diagnosed with colorectal cancer. He was scheduled to go through chemotherapy, radiation, and surgeries. I was working toward my bachelor's degree in psychology at the time while working as a massage therapist. I got my license in 2007. But after my dad's diagnosis, I stopped working toward my degree and helped keep his classes and his construction company going.

However, he never stopped going, teaching, or moving. Two days after his surgery in 2015, he had my older brother drive him ninety minutes away to watch me perform for my black belt test. He wanted to be the one to place the belt on me.

As with my "alternative" childhood, my father also turned to alternative medicine. Research Studies is my favorite subject in the world. Psychology research specifically, but my dad turned to me for his research needs, although he did some of his own too.

By this time, cannabis studies had been linked to treating cancer, but Ohio hadn't yet legalized medical cannabis use. Well, helping my father battle cancer was reason enough for me. So, we set to work.

He used a couple of other alternative medicines too. I know he'd be upset if I did not mention his raw aloe plants. He swears it's the best for radiation burns.

It was a long four-year battle of chemo, radiation, illness and cannabis, and thankfully, my dad beat his cancer. He's the strongest man I know. However, beating cancer isn't always the end of the story. He still has some health issues and pain every day. And it did not take long for my dad to get his medical card when Ohio passed medical cannabis use. It was a celebratory day in my house when my dad could get his medicine legally.

My dad is currently seventy-three and still teaching martial arts. As part of the martial arts, he's teaching kids self-confidence and emotional control and to keep working for their goals. I still help.

*****

Covid and Cannabis

Mother's Day weekend, 2020, I got covid in the most horrible way. I blame my taste in boyfriends! Unfortunately, my track record has not been so great. We dated just before the pandemic and just long enough for me to get covid. It was the original strain. I was really sick for thirty days. The whole world was on lockdown. We were told to not leave our house and make telemedicine appointments. I had gone to a drive-through testing site for my diagnosis. About three weeks in, I got a call that my covid test was lost. I was put on a waiting list for telehealth.

My dad became my hero again. "Call that cannabis doctor you know."

I met Dr. Bridget in January 2020, and it was then that I started learning more about the medical benefits of cannabis and the difference between CBD, CBN and the THC that society associates with cannabis. And I had tried Green Harvest Health freeze cream and body butter.

I scheduled an appointment and got in within a couple days. I have chronic pain from a car accident in 2017, and inflammation from covid was making it worse. I got my medical card while in quarantine for covid and became an official medical cannabis patient.

When I finally got my telemedicine appointment with a doctor who did not know me at all, he said to assume the test was positive, and since it had been three weeks, I could leave quarantine. I explained all the symptoms I still had, my main concern at that point being that I had severe eye infections. My eyes were oozing, inflamed, and bright red. "You can leave quarantine and go back to work," he repeated, even though I insisted I was still sick and stressed the concern with my eyes. Still, "You're good," was his closing advice.

Since I touch people for a living, I decided I would never go back to work looking like I had pink eye and would wait another couple of weeks. Covid was so new that no one truly knew much about it.

I eventually went back to work, but people were so scared, and the place where I worked wasn't busy. It was part-time at first, and there were no appointments. As appointments did finally start coming in—that was in late summer—I started having weird symptoms.

My eyes got better and hurt less as time went on. But the worst was "covid toe." These are blisters and lesions that develop on the toes of covid patients. Only for me, it was my fingers and toes. And as a massage therapist, I can't work without my hands. Steroid cream from the doctor didn't help. Eczema cream didn't help. I ended up leaving my job because I didn't know how to heal it.

While I had tried CBD in the past, I didn't really notice an effect. Learning more, I realized it's something you must take consistently before you feel the effects. So, I tried full-spectrum gummies. After that, I had no more painful blisters between my toes or my fingers. And I could work!

I'd still have weird muscle and joint swelling randomly. Mostly coinciding with my menstrual cycle. Every morning and night, my finger and feet joints would swell. It would stop when I started moving and stop when I was done. This went on until December 2021. I could still work, still practice martial arts, but I was in pain. I got my second vaccine, and it went away almost overnight.

Long covid/post covid wasn't known at this time. Doctors that I went to had no idea and said so. They didn't try to help. Covid clinics had just started being opened. And with January 1st, 2022, came round two!

My dad got a call that he had been around someone with active covid three days before. By that evening, three of us in my household tested positive. The initial infection was mild. I kept expecting the wild thirty-day ride as before. Nope, I went back out into the world after the quarantine period.

Two weeks later, I went to the ER. My vision was going in and out. I literally couldn't see—everything was blurry. My head was pounding. Any exposure to light was painful. I was treated like I was crazy, not in pain, and asked if I wanted to watch TV. I had to explain to the nurse that the light from the TV was painful to look at. I wasn't believed, mainly because light sensitivity is an autism trait.

While I knew I had autism, I couldn't afford an assessment before the pandemic. I paid for my autism diagnosis in April 2022. From my online adult autism communities, I've learned I'm not the only one with covid long-hauler symptoms.

I'm still scheduling with neuro-ophthalmologists. My vision has been steadily declining since May 2020 from chronic dry eye. Now, when I hit an autism burnout, my eyes shake. I'm also currently getting acupuncture.

Last week, my doctor put acupuncture needles in my eye sockets. It helped calm the nerves. While cannabis has helped to level out my covid leftovers, it's also helped with my sensory sensitivities, anxiety, appetite, sleep and more.

As I'm writing this, I'm making one of the biggest adjustments of my life. I'm shifting to work more at home and less outside of the house. My eyes and energy levels just keep draining. For the last six months, I've been setting up an online store and will be starting to take virtual one on one appointments for bodywork coaching. I'll still be doing massages and teaching martial arts, just not as much. While it's a difficult change, I'm looking forward to helping more people like me and spending more time at home.

I've lived most of my life with the stigma of being a "stoner" just because of who my father is. Even when I didn't touch cannabis. I still get it when I mention CBD or cannabis.

Nevertheless, alternative medicines and traditions are my passion, and I still plan to eventually get my Ph.D. in psychology research focused on mind/body alternative medicines like massage, martial arts, acupuncture, energy work, herbal medicine, and cannabis.

My dad is my hero. Cannabis has been medicine for us both. It's time to break the stigma. Educate people.

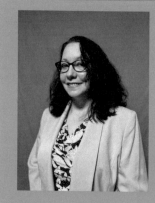

Rebecca Stanforth
Owner of Stone Path Studio
www.stonepathstudio.net
becca@stonepathstudio.net

Learn more about Rebecca
at www.courageincannabis.com:

How HIV Saved My Life: Turning Tragedy into Testimony
By Nicole Buffong

M s. Buffong, you are HIV positive."
This statement changed my life forever. I did not know it at the time, but being diagnosed with HIV in March of 2017 at the age of thirty-five was my biggest challenge and biggest blessing.

With my father being a Rasta man that healed his prostate cancer using an ital food plan, cannabis and noni juice, I knew there was a path to healing for my diagnosis as well. I was familiar with Dr. Sebi, Queen Afua and Dr. Africa and their work to reverse disease using diet. I discovered Minorities for Medical Marijuana in May of 2017, and by August, I met with the founder, Roz McCarthy and launched the State Chapter in Georgia in December.

Minorities for Medical Marijuana is an international non-profit organization that has twenty-seven chapters nationwide and five chapters internationally in the UK, Puerto Rico, Canada, Jamaica and Belize. Minorities for Medical Marijuana (M4MM) envisions a forward-thinking and progressive approach to social justice and equality in cannabis.

Through M4MM's commitment to education, public policy legislation, and outreach on issues important to diverse communities, we hope to promote global citizenry that will encourage the spirit of inclusivity in cannabis. For the next year and a half, I led the chapter in Georgia, learning how to be an advocate for patients and champion safe access to medicine.

I launched my brand and podcast, *Cannabis Connection World*, in January 2018 to educate my community on the basics of advocating and the research and science that helps us to understand how the cannabis plant reacts in our bodies.

By the end of 2018, my anxiety and paranoia had grown to levels that were detrimental to my health. Living in a state where I did not have access to safe medicine and being the voice and face of advocating for patients to use the cannabis plant was becoming a threat to my freedom and well-being. I found myself forced to become a medical refugee, and I had to leave Georgia.

In January 2019, I was asked to speak at a legalization rally in Trinidad and Tobago with the support of a brand marketing firm, AURA Ventures, which recruited me to be Director of Business Development in the Caribbean. AURA's home office is in Nevada, so I decided on Las Vegas.

In April 2019, I launched the state chapter for M4MM in Nevada. I began immersing myself in the cannabis community in the city. In October 2020, a new non-profit organization was established led by women advocates, The Chamber of Cannabis. I have sat on its board for the last three years. The Chamber of Cannabis is an industry trade association advocating for a conscientious, inclusive, and thriving industry in Nevada.

In January 2021, I accepted a role with M4MM that put me in charge of building chapters in eight states in the western region. Then, in February 2021, M4MM partnered with The Chamber of Cannabis to lobby for the consumption lounge bill in Nevada. Because of our efforts, social equity was mentioned in state statutes for the first time in Nevada.

Over the next two years, I recruited new leadership in the eight states and helped to educate my community on legislation that affected them and how they could become a part of the legal billion-dollar global industry.

In July 2021, I was also asked to serve on the board of directors for Association for Health Equity and Medicine (ACHEM). ACHEM [ay-kem] is a mutual benefit professional medical association for BIPOC healthcare professionals and students active or interested in cannabinoid medicine and health equity.

With ACHEM, I serve on a committee focused on providing education to the governments and resources to empower the people of the Caribbean and Africa to become a part of the thriving legal cannabis and hemp industry.

In 2022, I launched Purple Plant Magic, LLC. As a consulting firm, I advise individuals on how to become plant medicine advocates and business owners and how to find their lane in the billion-dollar global legal cannabis industry.

Most recently, in January 2023, I accepted an executive role within the organization as National Community Program Director, managing our ten national programs that serve our community and those most negatively impacted by the prohibition of cannabis for the last ninety years.

My journey to finding my purpose and healing over the last five years was because of that diagnosis of HIV. Cannabis saved my life in more than one way, and my passion for using plants as medicine has translated into a very promising career.

If you are canna-serious or canna-curious, today is the day to learn more about the layered cannabis industry. If you want to learn more about how to use cannabis as medicine or want to learn how to become a part of the budding industry, join the bandwagon. Minorities for Medical Marijuana has a free membership level, so become a part of our family and get all the information and resources you need to grow.

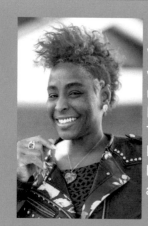

Nicole Buffong
Western Regional Director, M4MM
www.purpleplantmagic.com
nicole@purpleplantmagic.com
IG: @purpleplantmagic
Twitter: @purpplantmagic
Facebook: Nicole Buffong
Learn more about Nicole
at www.courageincannabis.com:

Higher Education Saved My Life

By Andrea Chaillet

***Content Advisory: This chapter will discuss experiences of rape, sexual assault, and eating disorders. Please engage in self care as you read this chapter.

1 in 6 women in the US are victims of attempted or completed rape. The age group 18-24 is at the highest risk. More than 50% of college sexual assaults occur in either August, September, October, or November (Rape, Abuse, and Incest National Network).

In 2018, I was raped the day before my second year of college. I was a few weeks shy of my 19th birthday. It was not the first time I had been sexually assaulted but it was the most traumatic occurrence. I am the 1 in 6.

In a state of shock, I tried hiding the situation from my friends and my family. However, suffering in silence got more difficult as my symptoms of PTSD got worse. I had frequent panic attacks, sometimes multiple times per day. I hid my body in oversized t-shirts and sweatpants even in the heat, not only to prevent people from sexualizing my body but also to hide the fact I was losing weight from not eating. It was getting difficult for me to focus in school because my brain was wracked with flashbacks, anxiety, and suicidal thoughts. I was lethargic all the time because I either slept all day or I had horrible insomnia that kept me up for days at a time. I wanted to escape reality by sleeping all day but often the nightmares and insomnia ruined my plans. I stopped going out with friends and to concerts because I couldn't be around crowds or loud noises.

Prior to the assault I was a straight A student from grade school through freshman year of college. Learning and being successful in school were always my top priorities. Now my brain and body's priorities were basic survival. I felt like a prisoner in my own body. By the summer of 2019 I realized that I would not mentally or physically be able to survive without getting professional help. I didn't have a lot of money and I didn't have good insurance. I remembered a business card from a local organization that I got when I performed in The Vagina Monologues at school. Due to my low income, Women Helping Women was able to connect me with a free support group and provide me with free individual therapy. Because of my symptoms and my experiences, I was diagnosed with PTSD. While I was trying to get my life back, this diagnosis felt like a death sentence. It made it feel like this was something that I would carry with me permanently and that it wouldn't get better. Only part of that was correct.

My therapist created a holistic treatment plan for me. I did not want to take pharmaceuticals to control my anxious and depressive symptoms. I started taking probiotics and vitamins every day to increase my mood. I began using essential oils to help me relax at home. I started meditating and doing yoga more often. Most importantly, my therapist wrote me a recommendation letter for medical marijuana.

The medical marijuana program in Ohio was fairly new when I was trying to obtain my card. I didn't know how or where to start the process. Luckily one of my friends had just gotten their card and recommended a clinic. My mom accompanied me on the day of my appointment. I could not stop shaking on the way there because I didn't know what to expect. Since I had a diagnosis and a recommendation letter from my therapist, my visit with the recommendation doctor was very simple. I discussed my symptoms and the doctor concluded I was a good candidate for MMJ. The clinic made sure I had a packet on how to register with the Board of Pharmacy and a list of dispensaries. The whole process took 20 minutes or less.

I wasn't given much information on what products would best treat my symptoms. I hadn't used any cannabis products before, not even CBD. I was completely lost and clueless when I walked into the dispensary for the first time. I panicked at the counter but the budtender took the time to ask what kind of relief I was looking for. My mom wanted to commemorate my first dispo visit by taking a picture of me with my bag outside the dispensary.

It took trial and error to find products that worked well for me and where to get them at an affordable price. As I experimented with different options, my quality of life increased. I was able to not only function better for work and school, but I got back to the activities that I loved. I registered with Accessibility Resources to help me complete my degree at The University of Cincinnati. With my accessibility agreement I was able to excuse myself from class for a few minutes to hit my vape to reduce the over-stimulation. I had less frequent panic attacks because I could take a few puffs whenever I started to get anxious. Medical marijuana also increased my appetite and my desire to enjoy cooking again.

I was able to live the "normal" life of a pre-pandemic college student. I started going to parties and concerts with my friends again. I became close friends with my neighbors, which is how I met my partner. Not living in fear helped me become a good friend and romantic partner again. I had ruined several friendships during my mental health struggles, and I'm lucky to have had a second chance to rebuild those connections.

When I changed my major in spring 2020 to environmental studies I was looking for a certificate that would pair well with it. I decided on horticulture. I remembered seeing a poster for Intro to Hemp and Medical Cannabis, which counted towards my certificate. When it came time to enroll in fall classes I registered for Intro to Hemp. I was extremely fortunate to have Sue Trusty as my instructor for it. The class, even though it was online, was such a bright spot for me during the pandemic. Sue's passion for the topic was contagious. One of my favorite projects was designing a grow facility, including irritation, lighting, and ventilation. I also enjoyed the weekly assignment of reading a cannabis-related article and reporting what was going on in the industry to my peers. Because of Sue, I got excited about reading *Cannabis Business Times*.

Sue announced plans for a Cannabis Studies Certificate, and shared a few details from her proposal with my class. I was one of the first students to apply for it when UC approved it. A lot of the curriculum coincided with my horticulture classes, which made it much easier for me to complete. I was even in a photoshoot to help market the new certificate.

In summer 2020 I enrolled in Hops and Hemp Field Experience, which further increased my interest in working in the cannabis industry. I was part of the first group of students to take this class. We set up a hop yard and a small hemp field at the UC Center for Field Studies. In addition to tending to our hops and hemp plants, we went on field trips. The most impactful field trips for me were the cannabis growth and processing facilities. I developed an interest in marijuana horticulture and processing. At the end of the summer we harvested the hemp and celebrated Sue's retirement.

Before Sue left UC, she had encouraged my class to enter an essay scholarship contest. I later found out that I was her only student who applied. The prompt was simple: describe one way to improve the cannabis industry. I knew I wanted to incorporate knowledge I had learned from my major in environmental studies, and I was inspired by my Sustainable Development class. In my paper I described how the cannabis industry can better fit the United Nations' Sustainable Development Goals from cultivation to post-consumer stages. This includes resource conservation, waste reduction, and social issues such as reducing the impact of the War on Drugs. I submitted my essay at the end of summer 2020 and received some of the best news in spring 2021! I was selected as a Veriheal Innovation in Cannabis Scholarship Award Winner! I was one of twenty undergraduate students from across the U.S. who received the honor. Not only was I featured on the Veriheal website, but I also received scholarship money that helped me complete my education. I'd like to think I helped put UC on the map for its cannabis studies curriculum.

The Veriheal scholarship led me to meet the woman who would mentor me through the rest of college and beyond. Bonnie Rabin had replaced Sue Trusty as the instructor for Intro to Hemp after her retirement. She reached out to me via email in fall 2021 to ask me to speak to her class to give advice on their Veriheal scholarship applications. I have since spoken to her class again about the scholarship and my current role in the cannabis industry.

Bonnie also invited me to attend the monthly Cincinnati Medical Marijuana Meetup that she hosts at a local brewery. These meetups allowed me to network with industry leaders while I was in school. I mingled with doctors, advocates, patients, dispensary managers, budtenders, cultivators, processors, and more. The cannabis community in Ohio is very supportive. At my first meetup I took notes on my phone of the career advice people gave me. In October 2022 I attended my first meetup as an industry worker instead of as a patient and a student.

After 5 long years, I finally graduated from The University of Cincinnati in spring 2022. I would not have been able to accomplish this without cannabis. It saved my life by regulating my symptoms of PTSD. It also gave me a sense of purpose. I was fortunate to attend one of the few universities that offers a cannabis-related curriculum.

A significant amount of sexual assault survivors drop out of school. Not only can assault cause lasting emotional damage, but it also impacts the victim's financial stability. Many quit or are forced to leave their jobs as they cope with symptoms of emotional distress (Maryland Coalition Against Sexual Assault). I am eternally grateful to my grandpa who helped me pay my tuition as I tried to rebuild my life. I am also thankful for the financial assistance I received from Veriheal. My mom, my friends Jordan and Marie, and my partner Donaven have all held me while I had flashbacks and panic attacks. At times they have forced me to eat and get out of bed. I would not have survived without their support.

For a few months after graduation I faced a few obstacles finding a job in the cannabis industry. Open positions were either too far away or didn't pay enough. I even got a talent manager from The United Green to scout out jobs for me. I decided to shoot my shot with a local business near UC. I interviewed for the Cincinnati location of The Eastern Kentucky Hemp Company, which is a hemp dispensary and dab bar. I was offered a position on the spot for a dispensary technician (aka budtender), and was quickly promoted to the general manager after about a month.

Because it is located close to UC, I interact with mostly college-aged young adults. My favorite aspect of my job is how much we bring to the community, especially in a state that has not legalized recreational use. Not everyone can afford to travel out of state to get the dispensary experience, so we strive to recreate it as much as possible. It is also the only dab bar in Ohio. The dab bar is a relaxed place for people to study, play board or video games with their friends, and watch movies. We host events like movie nights and Mario Kart tournaments. In a college area it is imperative for young people to have the option of lab-tested, quality products. You know exactly what you're getting without the risk of contamination by other substances. It's not enough to simply carry those products. There has to be education behind it too. I enjoy breaking down the misconceptions about Delta 8, explaining the differences between hemp and marijuana, and describing how THC-O is different from Delta 8.

Ultimately cannabis has brought me a lot of healing and peace. Combined with therapy, it allows me to function almost as well as I did before developing PTSD. It helped me realize that my life isn't over. Now I get to advocate for its medicinal benefits. Most importantly, I get to work directly in the Cincinnati cannabis community that helped me on my healing journey.

***If have suffered from sexual assault help is available:
Call 800.656.HOPE (4673) to be connected with a trained staff member

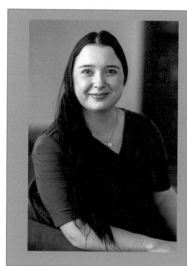

Andrea Chaillet
andrea@chaillet.org
IG: @chai.andie
LinkedIn: Andrea Chaillet

Learn more about Andrea
at www.courageincannabis.com:

EDUCATION SECTION

Why Am I A Cannabis Clinician

By Lynn Parodneck, MD

I remember staring up at the fluorescent beach mural as my left breast was exposed to thirty-five rounds of radiation over several weeks.

That first day, the tears flowed as I lay still awaiting the zap. I had been diagnosed with LCIS and DCIS, carcinoma in situ with a low propensity for progression. I can tell you what the backs of my clinician's heads looked like. I have little recollection of their faces due to their devotion to their computers. My journey as a patient had begun.

With each passing week, the fatigue pushed harder. I remember thinking if I had a bit of marijuana, this would be so much easier. I knew my college-aged sons had some in their rooms. Still, I could not ask them to go "shopping" for me. If they had been arrested, it would have been my fault.That was in 2012. Within two years, it would be legalized in New York for medical patients. Medical marijuana dispensaries opened in New York in 2016, and the recreational rollout in 2022.

I took the New York State four-and-a-half-hour course with literally crossword puzzles as part of the testing. This "course" is what determined if I could make cannabis recommendations.

I then contacted a few shops and toured the Vireo dispensary in White Plains. After deciding this was something I could do, I printed business cards and started reading. This subject was not part of medical school education. There was no official textbook, and research was limited. I applied physiology and common sense to figure out these puzzles. I spoke daily to Aashna, a pharmacist at Vireo.

My phone started ringing. Friends referred friends. I became a local conversation piece at Saturday night dinners. A few local doctors were interested in what this was about. I spoke at libraries, Rotary Clubs, and Lions Clubs events. Patients who knew me by my married name West were knocking on my door and were shocked to discover I had another alias. I became Dr. Lynn West to the cannabis community or Dr. Lynn West, "the cannabis doc."

Now retired from obstetrics, which is such a unique medical field, my view of health and wellness changed in this new space of cannabis. I realized that it was not only diseases that impacted the quality of life. Sleep, loss of appetite, pain, and nausea are all unpleasant states. With time, I began to see results. Patients began to feel better. Often, they figured out interesting product combinations and sequencing to give themselves an improved quality of life.
My practice started with patients suffering from chronic pain, Parkinson's, cancer, and migraines. It is my patients and their outcomes that amaze me. The longer I manage patients, their efforts and outcomes are truly surprising.

JF is a thirty-six-year-old EMT with PTSD. He was having visions of bleeding bodies and ghastly trauma. Unfortunately, alcohol became his solution until his wife found eleven empty bottles under the couch. He was obese and had tremors in his hands when it was time for his next drink. We spoke about vaping and how this could head off the "deep dive" before it took over. He found a seven-minute rock and roll guitar solo that he plays loudly on his phone when he vapes. Now, the song alone can settle him down when he knows this force from within is knocking on his door. He credits cannabis for turning him around.

I did a house call for a stroke patient. After eight years of quadriplegia, nobody wanted to be in the same room as Emily. She did not understand how her attitude and verbal abuse drove her adult children out of the family home. The first time I saw her, she called me "Bitch." Then I became "Lady," And soon after, "Lady Doctor" became my salutation. I suggested a high THC formulation to decrease muscle spasms and work as a mood elevator. This change in her demeanor was so remarkable her adult children became involved in her life again. For the first time in forever, Emily was pleasant, enjoyable and loving. I attended her wake and was inundated with hugs from family members. They knew cannabis brought their mom back, if only for a short period of time.

Bill had been dying for six and a half years. He was at his office in the Twin Towers in New York when the planes hit on 9/11 and successfully guided his team out of the tower, then ran to a friend's apartment in Chelsea. Seventeen years later, he developed a cough that worsened daily. After a year of this, he changed physicians and was diagnosed with lung cancer. He described the pain as "shards of glass eating away my chest." Bill wanted to get off the opioids administered by Hospice Care. He claimed that they made him nauseous, constipated, and loopy. He did not like "getting high." He claimed to be more of a "Martini Guy." His family had had enough of this waiting game. After he stopped using opioids, his erections returned. His wife was not excited by this and requested that I not come back.

These stories amaze me daily. Helping patients to reduce their medications-psych meds, opioids, and sleeping pills is a lofty ambition. When done correctly, with clean products under the supervision of a competent, licensed and knowledgeable individual, the results can be transformative. Why this is not legal in all fifty states and territories is baffling.

It has been proven that cannabis is *medicine*. If this medicine is reclassified by the DEA, medical insurance companies will be required to cover this expense and make these programs accessible to patients.

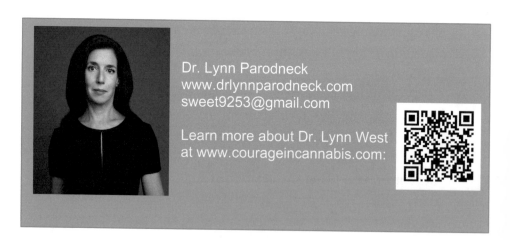

Dr. Lynn Parodneck
www.drlynnparodneck.com
sweet9253@gmail.com

Learn more about Dr. Lynn West
at www.courageincannabis.com:

Listening To The Song Of Cannabis

By Uwe Blesching, Ph.D.

A fter reading thousands of scientific papers on the herb's medicinal properties, I believe if cannabis had a song, its lyrics would be, "Balance is an easier, softer, and gentler way of being."

Life in the modern world is characterized by burnout, stress, and constant overwhelm. Rather than finding a natural rhythm that works for us, we become pressured to do more, be more, and achieve more.

When navigating life's challenges, balance can be a guiding light. However, balance, particularly in later life, is one of the most challenging things to achieve and the easiest to lose. This is why younger people typically bounce back from a cold, an injury, or other damaging events more quickly than older ones.

The gentle reader may wonder what this has to do with cannabis, and I say, consider this:

The human body has a natural system that produces cannabis-like chemicals. It is called the endocannabinoid system (ECS). This system aims to help keep our bodies balanced and healthy. These cannabis-like chemicals (the endocannabinoids) are like tiny messengers traveling around the body and telling the ECS how to maintain or re-establish balance. These endocannabinoids bind to unique places called receptors, which help the ECS know how to respond. So, the human body naturally produces its version of cannabis to help us stay balanced, stay healthy, and feel good!

However, as we age, it becomes harder for our bodies to maintain balance and stay healthy. This is partly because our bodies don't make as many endocannabinoid receptors as they used to. When we don't have as many receptors, our body can't work as well to recover from stress or damage. So, the older we get, the harder it is for our body to stay balanced and healthy because we have a weakened endocannabinoid system. This can make us more vulnerable to developing chronic diseases and long-term illnesses that can be very serious.

The proper use of cannabis can compensate for losing our ability to maintain or regenerate balance as efficiently as when we were young, healthy, and resilient. Indeed, recent research has demonstrated that many cannabis ingredients work together to bring about balance, which in return helps the body heal itself and become stronger.

When the right type of cannabis is used at the right dose and in the most appropriate form, it can provide three broad benefits for overall wellness.

First, it can help a person to relax deeply. Whether it's work pressure, family responsibilities, or personal issues, tension and stress can creep up on us unexpectedly and wreak havoc on our mental and physical health. In such moments, prioritizing relaxation for physical and psychological well-being is more important than ever. Not only does relaxation benefit our bodies, but it also helps to clear our minds and improve our ability to focus and make better decisions. In short, deep relaxation is a crucial component of self-care in these challenging times and should be prioritized as a necessary part of our daily routine.

Second, a therapeutic cannabis experience can make it easier to feel happy and positive. Happiness and positivity have a direct impact on our health and well-being. When we are happy, our brain releases endorphins, natural chemicals that promote pleasure and well-being. These endorphins also help reduce stress and anxiety, leading to a more robust immune system and a lower risk of chronic illnesses. Additionally, being positive and happy can help to increase resilience, which is our ability to cope with and bounce back from difficult situations. A positive mindset allows us to see challenges as growth opportunities rather than insurmountable obstacles.

Third, in the right setting and with positive intentions, cannabis-based products can help us feel a sense of "flow" in our thoughts and emotions. Achieving a sense of "flow" can profoundly impact our health and well-being. When we can let go of emotional baggage and enter a state of flow, we experience a sense of ease and inner harmony that can positively affect our physical, mental, and emotional health. This state of flow allows us to fully engage in the present moment, releasing us from the constraints of past traumas or future worries. By being fully present and engaged, we are better equipped to manage stress, anxiety, and other negative emotions. In addition, being in a state of flow can also boost creativity, productivity, and an overall sense of happiness and fulfillment.

These broad and general benefits of the medicinal use of cannabis can help everyone, especially patients challenged with chronic conditions.

Take, for instance, patients with post-traumatic stress disorder (PTSD). Therapeutic cannabis experiences can help patients relax, feel positive, and be present with all their emotions, including those that are painful, overwhelming, or dreadful, without using coping mechanisms like negative self-talk or aggression.

Another example includes seniors, the fastest growing group of patients new to cannabis as medicine, especially when dealing with chronic pain. More and more seniors with long-standing aches are unhappy about the limiting results, cost, and risks that come with the use of prescription drug painkillers.

Encouraged by studies that have shown that switching to cannabis-based therapeutics can effectively address chronic pains, safer and less expensively than opioids, more and more seniors are asking their treating physicians if cannabis is a possible option.

However, even though frustrated with the lack of progress and searching for better approaches, especially when treating chronic pain, many seniors still have reasonable concerns. Some may shun the idea of a remedy that could impair basic mental activities, increase the risk of falls, or produce a panic attack.

But there is good news on this front. New treatment options have come to light that we can use to alleviate all these concerns.

Here are some practical examples of what I mean that the reader may find helpful.

Any drug has the potential to produce a therapeutic or adverse effect. The same is true for cannabis, which is neither dangerous nor benign, especially compared to opioids. However, most of the dangers commonly reported about the use of cannabis can be laid at the feet of one specific cannabis ingredient called tetrahydrocannabinol (THC). What is important to know here is that cannabis contains hundreds of other components, many of which have proven to work to support balance as well as reduce many other common signs and symptoms, including those of chronic pain. One of the most well-known, intensively studied, and effective ingredients is cannabidiol (CBD).

Know that not all cannabis is the same. Some types of cannabis contain little or no THC. One of these works so well that it is available as an FDA-approved prescription drug called Epidiolex. It is given safely to children with severe epilepsy for whom the usual medicines are ineffective. This kind of cannabis is taken without the risk of getting tipsy, intoxicated, or anxious.

There is one caveat I should mention. An annual supply of the prescription version costs thousands of dollars. However, anyone with a small garden or a large pot full of good soil can grow Charlotte's web, a readily available unique cannabis flower containing primarily CBD, thus being virtually identical to Epidiolex.

Furthermore, new treatment options supporting a fully functioning endocannabinoid system go beyond using cannabis-based products. Exciting research results show that dietary changes, exercise, certain herbs, and even mindfulness techniques can support and restore an ailing ECS and our capacity to achieve balance in individual cells, tissues, organs, organ systems, and by extension, the whole self.

To describe them all goes beyond the scope of this chapter, but I wanted to share at least three proven approaches that you can find almost anywhere and use with the blessing of most government policies and control.

In recent years, mind-body approaches have gained traction as effective methods for improving overall health and well-being. One notable aspect of this holistic approach is its ability to enhance endocannabinoid signaling. By incorporating practices such as meditation, yoga, prayer, and mindful breathing, individuals can actively engage their minds in fostering a healthier and more balanced internal environment. These practices reduce stress and promote relaxation by stimulating the production and release of endocannabinoids, which in turn can improve endocannabinoid signaling. As a result, individuals who actively practice mind-body techniques may experience an uptick in their overall health and well-being, as these practices work synergistically to support optimal endocannabinoid function. By embracing the power of mind-body approaches, we follow the gospel of the herb and unlock the potential for improved endocannabinoid signaling, paving the way for a happier, healthier, and more balanced life.

Turmeric, a golden-colored spice renowned for its numerous health benefits, has also been found to support an ailing ECS. This ancient spice contains an active compound called curcumin, which is responsible for its vibrant color and potent medicinal properties. In addition, curcumin has been scientifically proven to preserve and restore optimal endocannabinoid signaling. Thus, turmeric helps to support our body's natural ability to self-regulate, adapt to stress, re-establish balance, and maintain a healthy immune system. Incorporating turmeric into our daily diet is a simple yet effective way to promote harmony and support long-term health.

Probiotics, known as the "good bacteria," has various health benefits, including their ability to improve endocannabinoid signaling and balance. They are commonly available in fermented foods such as yogurt, sauerkraut and kimchi.

We can effectively enhance the system's performance by incorporating probiotics into our daily routine. The link between probiotics and the endocannabinoid system lies in the gut-brain axis, a communication pathway that connects the digestive system with the brain. Probiotics work this axis by producing essential neurotransmitters and enzymes, directly improving endocannabinoid signaling. In turn, this helps maintain balance in the body, leading to improved physical and mental well-being.

Essential fatty acids are the primary building blocks that make up the ECS. The human body does not make omega-3 fatty acids. We must consume them by eating fish, nuts, and seeds. Omega-3 essential fatty acids significantly contribute to the optimal functioning of the ECS by increasing the production of anti-inflammatory endocannabinoids. These compounds help to reduce inflammation, improve mood, and promote a healthy immune system. By incorporating omega-3-rich foods into your daily diet, we can effectively enhance the performance of our ECS, ensuring better overall health and well-being.

The Song of Cannabis preaches the importance of balance—a concept that resonates not only in the world of medicinal cannabis but in all aspects of life.

Consider embracing an easier, softer, and gentler way of being by incorporating CBD-rich cannabis, mindfulness, turmeric, probiotics, and omega-3s to reach for a healthier ECS and an overall sense of balance in body, mind, and spirit.

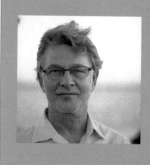

Uwe Blesching, PhD
Author of Cannabis Health Index
Founder of Cannakeys
www.uweblesching.com
uwe@cannakeys.com

Learn more about Uwe
at www.courageincannabis.com:

A Higher Appreciation
By Tyrone Russell

I approach this plant with care. I approach it with concern and with a sense of protection as if it has the capability to save lives and the ferociousness to take them. I approach it as if I've witnessed a white woman who was anti-cannabis resort to it as she tries to revive what is now a shell of her husband. I treat it with the respect it deserves because that plant has indeed worked for that woman, and while her husband will never be the same, his relationship with cannabis allowed him to shoot hoops with his grandchild in their New Jersey driveway, something he could not physically do for years.

I approach it with caution because the disrespect that folks have shown when all they see is profit while promoting a message of irresponsibility had my closest family members fighting damaging addiction at an early age.

I approach it as if it has single-handedly torn apart communities where I once lived, to the point where people from those communities only fear the power of God more than they do the potency of "weed."

I truly see the plant as medicine, whether used in adult-use spaces or medical markets. In fact, I appreciate those states that take their time in going "recreational" as they build out a medical market that sees a rise in patient counts and a decrease in deaths through overdose from opioids—the states that, as an industry, we complain about but should embrace more.

TYRONE RUSSELL

I treat the plant as if it can divide a personal relationship as fast as it can build a global economy. After all, this was the plant that I was selling when my mom sat me down and said she "heard a rumor." And with tears in her eyes, she begged me to stop because we couldn't lose everything she had come so far for as a single mom.

Anything that could bring my superhero mother to her knees has the power to lift her up, and I believe it.
This plant calms my mind. It puts my wife's anxiety to rest so she can sleep at night.

From topicals to suppositories, to gummies and pure flowers, we will continue to educate our communities from seed to the sell because we know that with this great plant power, a greater responsibility to handle it with reverence should be promoted and upheld with a higher appreciation.

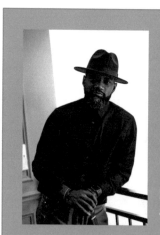

Tyrone Russell
President of Cleveland School of Cannabis
CEO of Faces International
www.Russellfe.com
tyronerussell@csceducation.com
IG: @tyrussell365
Linkedin: Tyrone Russell

Learn more about Tyrone
at www.courageincannabis.com:

Being Medical In A Recreational Culture

By Dr. Bridget Cole Williams

I grew up in a pharmaceutical tolerant environment. Whatever ailed my family, we took medicines for it. My grandmother was the matriarch who would suggest more holistic options, such as aloe vera, cod liver oil and tying salt pork to my foot when I stepped on a toothpick, and it broke off inside my foot. I did this multiple times. Don't ask. Otherwise, we were a medicine accepting family. Both my brother and I became physicians, not because we believed so heavily in Western medicine, actually the contrast. . We became physicians because my father died of cancer when I was twelve and my brother was seventeen. We were determined to do something about it.

My brother faced our pain directly. He is currently a hematologist/oncologist at Michigan State University. However, my father's illness impacted me differently. During numerous phases of his illness, we went to the hospital every evening to visit my giant of a father. A giant not in stature but in brilliance, eloquence and confidence. What I found confusing was the medical team. They bombarded the room in their white coats and stethoscopes, walking in six or eight people deep. They did not acknowledge my mother, brother or me. They did not see a family suffering as the head of our family was slipping away.

It was shocking to see how dismissive they were of my powerful yet silent father. Did they not know how majestic this man was? Every day they walked out of that

227

room, I would say to my mom, "I could do this so much better," and she would always respond, " And so you should."

I became a family medicine doctor and spent over fifteen years at the Cleveland Clinic. I developed a heart for the medical patient, their experiences and their struggle navigating the medical system. My mission was to be a safe place, an ally and an advocate to help patients in their wellness journey.

I entered the cannabis space because of one patient who suggested cannabis as an alternative to her diabetes medications. I doubted her, challenged her, and ultimately I was proven wrong. I was curious and provided support as I watched and assisted in her cannabis journey. I saw her health transform in a way pharmaceuticals were not doing. I realized I wanted to support patients in their journey and educate them on the tie between pharmaceuticals and how cannabis could support their wellness and possibly replace their prescription drugs.

The medical market dominated the U.S. cannabis market with a share of 77% in 2022.[1] Medical cannabis proved its significance despite the overwhelming presence of the recreational focus and products that are available. As of April 2023, thirty-seven states have medical cannabis programs, and twenty-one states have medical and recreational programs.[2] As more states develop cannabis

---

[1] https://www.grandviewresearch.com/industry-analysis/us-cannabis-market

[2] https://www.cnn.com/2023/04/20/us/states-where-marijuana-is-legal-dg/index.html

programs, more Americans are trying cannabis for the first time.

According to a YouGov poll, the percentage of U.S. adults who say they have tried marijuana is sitting at 52%, the highest measurement to date.[3] As the numbers grow and the market expands, the cannabis industry continues to focus on the recreational user who tends to pursue more THC as their "drug of choice."

However, medical patients have been a great deal of the catalyst for legalization. State programs have been approved on the backs of Charlotte Figi, Mary Jane Rathbun, Jack Herer, the Knox Docs, and many of the people and the stories shared in Courage in Cannabis Volumes One and Two. However, as recreational policies are accepted, the medical patient who once was so important gets lost.

You can argue that all cannabis shoppers are medical consumers, and I agree, for many, this is true. But the insufficient medical products that are available, the "get stoned" messaging and sparse consumer education suggests that medicine is not focal to the industry.

I do not at all demonize the euphoric experience of cannabis. I would much rather have Americans high at a wedding, bar or club than messy drunk, obnoxious and dangerous. People can experience cannabis however they choose, but the industry needs to put its money behind the research. Innovation and quality care are needed to change the lives of cancer, seizure, pain, mental health, autism and inflammatory bowel patients and many, many others. If we don't, then someone else will.

---

[3] https://today.yougov.com/topics/society/articles-reports/2022/04/07/half-of-americans-have-tried-marijuana

Pharmaceutical corporations are busy at work creating synthetic and plant-based products to not only compete with the plant-based cannabis industry but to surpass them. Despite the incredible distrust that has been built toward the American health system and pharmaceutical industry, they will have well-designed research, superior testing, specified dosing, insurance coverage and, most likely, the FDA on their side.

Dronabinol has been available for years, Epidiolex® was approved for pediatric seizures, and Idrasil® is now available in California. Big pharma will inevitably gain the medical health professionals. Yes, the same physicians and health institutions that say there is not enough research and they do not approve of this "illicit addictive drug" will readily be writing scripts for cannabis. They will also be providing a higher quality of care than the "card docs" who unscrupulously provide medical cannabis access with little to no patient guidance or care.

The sudden professionalism that these pharmaceutical-driven healthcare providers will provide, hopefully, will turn patients away from the quick card options and will challenge these card companies to provide higher-quality care. I was offered a job to be a "cash for cards" doctor, which I turned down because I believed patients deserved better. The future of medical cannabis will involve pharma and pharma alone if we are not careful.

Pharmaceutical cannabis will also be attractive to the medical cannabis patient community as well. Many patients are seeking relief from something and are lost between products that are too concentrated for some patients and feeling like they are doing something corrupt or immoral.

Reefer Madness is *alive*! The medical cannabis community is still trying to define itself and looking for support where the adult-use market knows itself well. Although welcoming to the medical patient, it can be confusing to that patient who is unsure if being a patient means they are a part of the culture and, honestly, trying to determine what the culture is all about. Whether they trust big pharma or not, their messaging is clear. They provide FDA-approved medications to sick people, and if you have insurance, they will accept that too!

Currently, my job is not to simply provide cards. Medical cards are the administrative part. My job is to be a guide and trusted resource. I am to provide my medical knowledge in a sometimes questionable and unregulated medical space. I am also here for other doctors. I build rapport with my patient's other physicians so they can have a cannabis specialist they can converse with so we make decisions for our patients together. My job is to watch out for my chronic consumers by asking the critical question, "Are you using cannabis, or is cannabis using you?™" As a result, I support them in tolerance breaks and building a healthy relationship with cannabis or encourage their sobriety when that is possible.

With the concentration of THC in products and flowers almost doubling from 2008 to 2017,[4] it is not surprising that the dependency rate of cannabis has also almost doubled from nine percent of people who use marijuana becoming dependent on it now rising to about

---

[4] https://www.cdc.gov/marijuana/health-effects/addiction.html

seventeen percent in those who start using in their teens.[5] It is my conviction that we protect our youth as we explore this new world of legal cannabis use. We have viewed excessive alcohol use on college campuses as a right of passage, but as dabs and other cannabinoid concentrates gain popularity, we can be facing new dependency and health issues we have not foreseen.

Cannabis is the miracle plant that just keeps giving. I support the safety, joy and creativity of adult use, and I am passionate about its medicinal healing. However, I implore the industry to not give up on the medical patient just because adult use is available or insight. Instead, keep your focus on what the plant actually provides:

- Hope for my bedridden 45 year-old multiple sclerosis patient.
- Relief for my 83 year-old severe arthritic patient.
- Freedom for my 50 year-old PTSD veteran patient.
- Comfort for my 32 year-old depression and anxiety patient.
- Peace for my 65 year-old cancer patient.
- Safety for my 26 year-old recovering opioid addiction patient.
- Life for my 3 year-old epileptic patient.

Cannabis is more than the "high." It is life for many. With knowledgeable doctors, superior research, and patient-friendly dispensaries, we can change a country filled with illness to a world of global wellness and sustainable resources.

---

[5] https://nida.nih.gov/publications/research-reports/marijuana/marijuana-addictive

The diversity of cannabis culture should always remain. The culture is rich with artists, intellectuals, musicians and more who explore their creativity through cannabis, dominating much of the narrative in popular music. It is also rich with scientists, medical professionals, researchers and shamen who explore the healing gifts of this plant. We can all exist together.

The plant is incredibly diverse, and so are we. No one aspect should overshadow the other. On the contrary, medical and adult use should provide support and perspective to one another as we continue to explore this journey called cannabis.

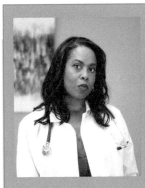

Dr. Bridget Cole Williams, MD
CEO of DrBridgetMD
Embody and ReclaimMD
www.DrBridgetMD.com
https://linktr.ee/DrBridgetMD

Learn more about Dr. Bridget
at courageincannabis.com:

Legacy To Leadership
By Michael Lawson Jr., MS

My journey in cannabis began in 1993 with the passing of Proposition 215. California legalized medical cannabis, and you could literally smell the excitement in the air.

I understood cannabis was medicine, but I admit it was a bit confusing initially. I saw my peers getting stoned and my elders coping with cancer and glaucoma. Although I knew it was medicine, I also saw people recreationally using the plant. My curiosity about the plant has taken me on a journey that required *Courage in Cannabis*.

In high school, I was an occasional smoker and a year-round athlete. When I arrived in Atlanta, Georgia, at Morehouse College, I began consuming cannabis on a consistent basis and started to understand the various medicinal benefits. I soon realized that cannabis was helping me cope with post-traumatic stress and anxiety.

During this period of discovery, I also had multiple encounters with law enforcement and became familiar with the State of Georgia and the City of Atlanta criminal justice system. I remember sitting in Fulton County jail thinking, I'm in jail over a gram of weed; how could this be? After my second encounter with the law, I continued to use cannabis and was steadfast in my belief that it is our human right to use this medicine.

Years later, my passion would shift into purpose when I received my Master of Science in Clinical Mental

Health Counseling from Mercer University. My journey seemed to have come full circle after spending fifteen years navigating the legacy market and studying medicinal cannabis.

In 2014, I found my purpose in the courtroom advocating for clients who faced prison time for cannabis consumption. My understanding of cannabis and mental health made me an asset to community members who found themselves in the crosshairs of the law only because they chose to use cannabis to improve their overall well-being.

Prior to the legalization of cannabis, there were not many education platforms that provided access to scholarly resources regarding cannabis science. As a therapist, this made my job more difficult when trying to articulate the importance of the Endocannabinoid system to community stakeholders.

After seeing a void in the cannabis education space, I founded Cannabis Media Collective, a platform that elevates cannabis science, empowers entrepreneurs, and educates citizens on how the cannabis plant can improve outcomes in multiple domains of physical and mental health.

I want to share my story with the world, encourage readers to pursue their passion, and be sure that such a pursuit benefits everyone we touch along the way.

Have courage in cannabis!

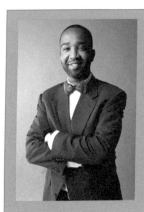

Michael Lawson Jr, MS
Cannabis Media Collective
www.cannabismediacollective.com
michael@cannabismediacollective.com

Learn more about Michael
at www.courageincannabis.com:

Redemption For Returning Citizens

By Dionne Dowdy-Lacey

At face value, the criminal justice system is a societal agreement to maintain law and order amongst its citizens. But, equally vital to our social contract is providing the opportunity for redemption for those who have accepted the consequences of their offenses. However, many formerly incarcerated individuals, especially Black and brown populations, continue to pay their debt to society long after they are released. And despite serving their sentences and showing signs of productivity, this debt becomes a never-ending burden signifying one message: that they will never be fully accepted back into society.

We can collectively agree that every American citizen deserves the right to liberty and justice. In that case, we must be willing to challenge our biases and preconceived notions reserved for our returning citizens. We cannot demand reformation yet strip them of their ability to support themselves, their families, and their communities, all while ostracizing them from the labor market. This, in turn, not only perpetuates recidivism but is counterproductive morally.

My name is Dionne Dowdy-Lacey, and I am the United Returning Citizens (URC) Executive Director, a 501c3 non-profit corporation serving the Tri-County and Youngstown area in Ohio.

My passion for reducing recidivism was born out of my own experience as the wife of my formerly incarcerated late husband. While he served his sentence, I learned firsthand the lack of support available to my family and others. My journey and those of the men and women who feel they are climbing a mountain with proverbial boulders on their backs drive my passion for this work. Their frustrations, motivation, resilience, and courage are daily affirmations to step in the gap on their behalf and rewrite the narrative. As such, URC has worked tirelessly for eight years to circumvent systemic biases that unequally hinder returning citizens who are not defined by their pasts but inspired by the possibility of creating a better future.

Through our URC Grows program, we lead the charge by facilitating opportunities in the emerging cannabis industry. For those we support, the cannabis sector is a clear path to education access, economic mobility, and social justice reform.

Why URC Grows Matters

If I had a magic eraser, I would wipe away years of miseducation around cannabis and its stigma in people's minds. From end to end, URC Grows is a program for agricultural experts in their field who happen to have a criminal background. For years, they have perfected their craft underground and now have the chance to positively showcase their knowledge to impact their communities and the cannabis industry at large.

Education

One of the primary challenges formerly incarcerated individuals experience is a lack of access to education, which significantly hinders their future career outlook. At every educational level, formerly incarcerated people are negatively and disproportionately impacted, leaving them vulnerable to higher unemployment rates. For instance, according to Prison Policy reports, formerly incarcerated individuals are more likely to have GEDs than traditional high school diplomas and are eight times less likely to graduate college than the general public. These grim stats are unacceptable and reveal the painful circumstances preventing people from living their desired lives. In an ever-evolving workforce, lacking the credentials to compete becomes a crippling roadblock that, left unaddressed, leads to recidivism.

The growing cannabis industry presents a significant uptick in skill development, and we understand that collaboration will expand our capacity to support our communities. We are grateful for the funding support we have been provided by the Hawthorne Social Justice Fund within The Scotts Miracle-Gro Foundation. It is through their support that we've established a partnership with Riviera Creek Holdings, a medical cannabis cultivator in Youngstown, and the Cleveland School of Cannabis, to launch our three-part program. URC Grows allows participants to earn an Ohio Department of Education-approved certification and entrepreneurial development. By the end of the program, students will be able to start their own grow or work with an URC-operated grow facility.

Limitless Economic Mobility

Bianca Pressley is a twenty-eight-year-old Youngstown native who is our first URC Grows graduate and is a stellar example of what happens when we empower returning citizens with the tools and resources they need to survive and thrive. Born with an innate interest in plants and recognizing their medicinal properties, she enrolled in URC Grows through our partnership with the Cleveland School of Cannabis Executive Program and has continued to excel. Upon graduation, Pressley launched two successful entrepreneurial endeavors, the "Governor's Garden" and "B. The Alchemist." Her companies provide health, nutrition, wellness coaching, and alternative holistic medical treatment.

At the end of 2021, Ohio's medical market generated nearly $500 million in sales, and projections are slated to continue an upward trend. On par with the U.S. cannabis market, which is expected to grow exponentially over the next few years, Ohio is positioned to become one of the leading states in the Midwest by 2025. If state lawmakers can pass adult-use legislation, the Buckeye State could create an even larger market with nearly nine million adults over the age of twenty-one.

Among those adults are thousands of returning citizens, like Pressley, who, given a chance, could establish livable wages and small enterprises as cannabis growers.

Cannabis Social Justice Reform

Reportedly, in 2019, the United States had 545,602 marijuana-related arrests and 500,395 possession-related arrests, a slight drop from 608,000 arrests in 2017, according to the FBI (www.freshwatercleveland.com). Additionally, of the 663,367 people arrested for cannabis in 2018, ninety-two percent of those detained resulted in drug possession charges. Black and Latino people were disproportionately targeted and represented forty-six point nine percent of those incarcerated, despite representing only thirty-one point five percent of the population.

While some states have legalized all uses of marijuana, eighty to ninety percent of the marijuana industry is operated and led by white owners (www.insider.com). This creates a disproportionate, unjust access issue for formerly incarcerated individuals. While some states and municipalities may eventually see their convictions overturned, it still leaves a barrier to entry into the emerging cannabis industry.

Furthermore, Ohio has legalized medical marijuana use and has severe restrictions on cultivating, processing and distributing medical marijuana. Licenses to grow, approach and sell were a very restrictive process and, to date, have all been distributed. That means new licenses are not being assigned at this time. More than twenty thousand Ohioans are arrested yearly for marijuana possession, www.freshwatercleveland.com. In 2018, twenty-one point two percent of formerly incarcerated individuals in Ohio remained unemployed, with a large proportion of those unemployed having marijuana possession as the charge. Overall, in Ohio, there is a tremendous need for policy reform.

Actionable Progress

Imagine running a competitive race as a professional athlete and right before the start being told that you must compete without any shoes. Although you could still run and possibly win, the disadvantage would significantly stifle your odds of success. Similarly, returning citizens, especially those with felony backgrounds, are restricted from fully participating in the cannabis business compared to the general public. Under the Ohio Administrative Code 3796:6-2, returning citizens with felony backgrounds related to controlled substances are disqualified from dispensary employment and a cultivating license, creating yet another obstacle they must face to partake in the sector. Although there are avenues for some returning citizens to gain access to a cultivating license by petitioning the State Board of Pharmacy, institutional bias presents a negative compounding effect for Black and brown growers, who are most denied compared to their white counterparts.

Evidence shows that it's highly probable marijuana will be removed from the federal narcotics classification lists. The United States House of Representatives has passed federal legislation that would decriminalize marijuana in totality and expunge the records of those incarcerated on marijuana distribution and possession charges, with many states already legalizing medical use and, in some states, recreational use.

I have watched returning citizens struggle through a system that has been negligent in its ability to care for and equitably protect them. We can no longer sit idle as portions of our communities are left out of the American dream without bearing the burden of their suffering.

Now is the time to act, push forward and hold up our end of the bargain so that everyone willing and capable can co-create the communities we all can be proud of.

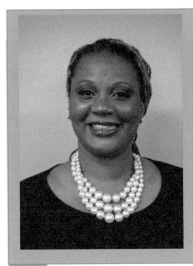

Dionne Dowdy-Lacey
Executive Director of United
Returning Citizens
www.unitedreturningcitizens.org
info@unitedreturningcitizens.org

Learn more about Dionne
at www.courageincannabis.com:

SPONSOR PROFILES

BLEV 614

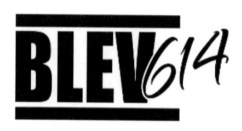

is a full audiovisual production company located in Columbus, OH. We are the ultimate solution for your end-to-end Video and Audio needs. Our primary areas of expertise are in providing quality, cost effective video and audio production, video distribution, promotion, and maintenance services to our clients.. From news, sports, entertainment, our production services expands across mobile, digital and social platforms. Our mission is to be a leader for Central Ohio's businesses in video production and web strategy by providing technical and creative solutions that fit each client's needs, while operating with professionalism and integrity. Victoria Ludaway, owner of BLEV 614 Network, currently produces a network TV show called Blev 614, airing on NBC4-WCMH.

To learn more, visit: www.blev614.com
BLEV614NETWORK@gmail.com
FB, IG, Tiktok: @Blev614network

Jade Sponsor

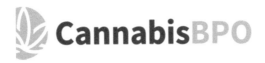

CannabisBPO is a specialty provider of contact center services for the cannabis industry with locations in the US and Canada. We provide inbound and outbound contact center services in a 24/7 environment. Our core service channels are phone, chat, mail, email, text, and social media for sales, customer service, and technical support projects. We help cannabis businesses drive sales and maintain brand integrity.

Our commitment to helping our clients achieve their goals is our core mission. Our unique blend of experience allows CannabisBPO to offer custom solutions that are tailored to each of our client's individual needs. Every program is strategically designed to help you achieve your goals and track your progress. Contact us today and discover how we can help you drive revenue and reduce operational costs.

To learn more, visit: www.cannabisbpo.com **Jade Sponsor**
www.linkedin.com/company/cannabisbpo/

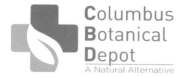

In 2013 Joseph Brennan lost both his father and his uncle back-to-back due to the complications of pharmaceutical-based medicine. Shortly thereafter, Joe came across a mainstream television documentary about a cannabis compound called Cannabidiol (CBD) being used to successfully treat children with seizures. It was at that moment he saw an opportunity to spread the word, help others, and bring this plant compound to the forefront of present awareness. In memory of his father he started vending shows and festivals around Ohio spreading the word about non-psychoactive, hemp-derived CBD. This evolved four years later into Columbus Ohio's first CBD only specialty retail/online store! We specialize in education on the endo-cannabinoid system (ECS), its functions, as well as the role plant-based (phyto) cannabinoids play in interacting with this important component of human and animal biology.

Jade Sponsor

To learn more, visit Columbus Botanical Depot online: www.cbdhemphealth.com
Joe is also an author in Courage in Cannabis Volume One. See more about
Joe at courageincannabis.com:

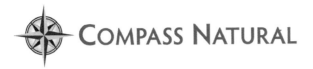 COMPASS NATURAL

Based in Boulder, Colorado, the "Epicenter of the Natural Products Industry," Compass Natural is a boutique digital marketing, branding, PR, and business development agency serving the rapidly growing market for natural, organic, socially responsible, eco-friendly and other healthy lifestyles products. Founded in late 2001 and driven by a commitment to create a better world through business, Compass Natural has been a leader in the Lifestyles of Health and Sustainability (LOHAS) market.

To learn more, visit: www.compassnaturalmarketing.com

Emerald Sponsor

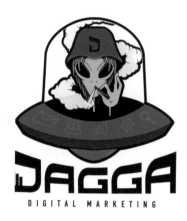

Dagga Digital Marketing is predicted on using education, data, technology, and media to expand the overall knowledge of cannabis medicine, lifestyle, and business in a creative way. The goal is to uplift small businesses and experts in order to help destigmatize cannabis. Adonis Fitzgerald, CEO of

2019. He is dedicated to
scale with digital marketi

admin@daggamarketing.
LinkedIn: Dagga Digital
Instagram: @daggadigita

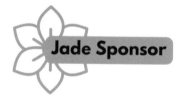

Jade Sponsor

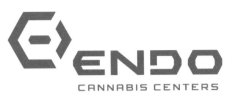

Endo Cannabis Centers were founded to be much more than a great place to buy premium-quality Cannabis products. We invite you to share in what we call the "Endo Vibe" and join us in becoming Endo Enthusiasts!

The Endo Vibe embraces a philosophy to serve as a proactive community partner that educates, uplifts, and makes a difference with positive actions to support and help our neighbors.

You'll feel the Endo Vibe when you visit our store, where you'll have access to premium-quality products and a chill shopping experience you can see, feel, and touch. Our Endo Experts will answer your questions and provide recommendations based on your needs and wants – your vibe, your way.

To learn more, visit: www.endovibe.com

info@endovibe.com

Instagram: @endo_vibe

Emerald Sponsor

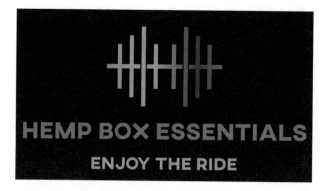

Hemp Box Essentials is Georgia's first modified shipping container hemp food truck. Our mission is to educate Georgians on hemp CBD health and wellness. CEO and Founder, Sandy Moore, has worked hard to establish relationships with local metropolitan advocates such as Peachtree NORML and Georgia Justice Project that assists individuals having difficulties acquiring employment because of a Georg expungement clinics.

Learn more go to: www.l
thehempboxetc@gmail.co
FB, IG, Twitter: @hempl

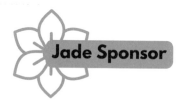

Jade Sponsor

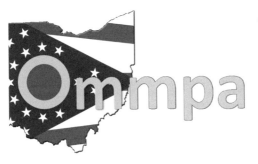

The Ohio Medical Marijuana Physicians Association (OMMPA) was formally established in May, 2019. Our mission is to provide information, representation, tools, and support to Ohio Medical Marijuana Physicians and their practices. While physicians are busy managing their practices, OMMPA provides extra capacity to work issues on their behalf with the Ohio State Medical Board and the Ohio State Pharmacy Board. OMMPA connects with professionals across the Medical Marijuana industry to help our members overcome the barriers they face, through education, scaled services, and channeling their collective voices. Our end goal is to ensure Ohio physicians are enabled to provide efficient care for their patients.

To learn more, visit: www.ommpa.com

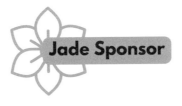

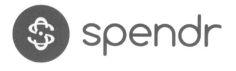 spendr

At Spendr, we've built a one-of-a-kind platform that combines payments, rewards, and marketing for cannabis. Our partner dispensaries can offer compliant and cashless payment options, along with Spendr-funded rewards. They're also able to engage with customers through integrated marketing tools across in-app, email, and push channels. Consumers can pay without fees or the hassle of cash, which means faster transactions and shorter lines.

Lucas Gould, our founder and CEO, is on a mission to be a leader in normalizing cannabis, starting by delivering a unique, secure, enjoyable, and rewarding experience for both cannabis consumers and dispensaries. Buying legal cannabis should be safer, easier, rewarding, and more "normal", and everything we do is in pursuit of that goal.

To learn more, visit: www.spendr.com/business
hello@spendr.com.

Instagram: www.instagram.com/getspe

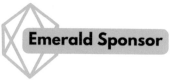

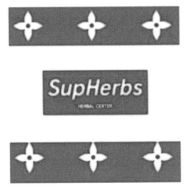

Supherbs Herbal Center was formed in mid 2018, with the passage of both Federally legal Hemp, and Michigan State legalizing cannabis recreationally. Our owner Mr. King has been consuming cannabis and hemp products since he was a late child, upon which he immediately noticed several benefits, both physically and mentally. Millions of people in our nation have success stories due to cannabis, whereas the so-called medicine the doctors push has little to zero effect, keeping the end user in a constant loop of dependency of a product that doesn't work, along with terrible side effects. Cannabis and hemp actually work! Thus, Supherbs Herbal Center was created, to bring the public not just THC, but rather all of the amazing compounds and their individual benefits. Mr. King owns Supherbs Herbal Center, Dank Bakes, Dapper Canna, and a few small nurseries, with the end goal of entering all legal markets, but keeping the legacy vibe.

To learn more, visit: www.shopsupherbs.com

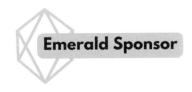

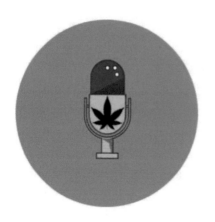

The Canna Mom Show was created to help crush cannabis stigma by sharing the voices and stories of the women breaking barriers and building businesses in the emerging cannabis industry, one canna story at a time. Joyce Gerber is a mother and a former family law attorney. Each week she interviews women from across the country and around the world who are pioneers in the cannabis health movement as caregivers and entrepreneurs.

To learn more, visit: www.thecannamomshow.com

Emerald Sponsor

Made in the USA
Columbia, SC
02 December 2024

47166161R00141